Current schi

Third edition

Editors
Martin Lambert, Dieter Naber
Department of Psychiatry and Psychotherapy
Center for Psychosocial Medicine, University Medical Center Hamburg-Eppendorf
Germany

Contributors
Eóin Killackey, Patrick McGorry
ORYGEN Research Centre
Department of Psychiatry, University of Melbourne, Victoria
Australia

Steffen Moritz, Ingo Schäfer, Britta Galling, Liz Rietschel
Department of Psychiatry and Psychotherapy
Center for Psychosocial Medicine, University Medical Center Hamburg-Eppendorf
Germany

Tim Lambert
Psychological Medicine, Concord Clinical School, University of Sydney
Australia

Philippe Conus
Department of Psychiatry
Centre Hospitalier Universitaire Vaudois and University of Lausanne
Switzerland

Frauke Schultze-Lutter, Benno Schimmelmann
Bern Early Recognition and Intervention Centre
University Hospital of Child and Adolescent Psychiatry Bern
Switzerland

Stephan Ruhrmann
Early Recognition and Intervention Center
Department of Psychiatry and Psychotherapy of the University of Cologne
Germany

🐎 Springer Healthcare

Published by Springer Healthcare Ltd, 236 Gray's Inn Road, London, WC1X 8HB, UK.

www.springerhealthcare.com

© 2012 Springer Healthcare, a part of Springer Science+Business Media.

First edition published in 2005
Second edition published in 2009

British Library Cataloguing-in-Publication Data.

A catalogue record for this book is available from the British Library.

ISBN 978-1-908517-46-3

Project editor: Alla Zarifyan
Designer: Joe Harvey
Artworker: Sissan Mollerfors
Production: Marina Maher
Printed in Great Britain by Latimer Trend

Contents

Biographies

Editors

Martin Lambert is a professor of psychiatry at the University of Hamburg, where he is the head of the Psychosis Center, which includes the Psychosis Early Detection and Intervention Center (PEDIC). He performed his psychiatric training at the Department of Psychiatry and Psychotherapy at the University Medical Center in Hamburg, Germany. During his training, he spent 2 years at the Early Psychosis Prevention and Intervention Centre (EPPIC) in Melbourne, Australia. Professor Lambert's current research interests include the pharmacological and psychosocial treatment of schizophrenic, bipolar, and first-episode psychosis patients, and, especially, aspects of integrated care, remission and recovery, quality of life, and subjective wellbeing. Professor Lambert is the head of the network for a better mental health in Hamburg, which was founded by the German Research Association. He is the editor and author of several books about schizophrenia and has published various articles on schizophrenia and first-episode psychosis.

Dieter Naber has been the director of the Psychiatric University Hospital in Hamburg, Germany, since 1995. After studying medicine in Göttingen and Bonn, Germany, Professor Naber worked at the Psychiatric Hospital of the University of Munich, Germany, from 1977 to 1995 as a ward doctor and then as a senior physician. In 1987, he gained a postdoctoral lecturing qualification with his lecture "The etiological and therapeutic significance of endorphins in endogenous psychosis." Professor Naber conducted research during two periods at the National Institute of Mental Health, in 1978–1980 and again in 1984–1985. His current research concentrates on long-term neuroleptic treatment, efficacy and side effects of second-generation neuroleptics, and the subjective effects of neuroleptics.

Contributors

Eóin Killackey is an associate professor and clinical psychologist at the ORYGEN Youth Health Research Centre and the Centre for Youth Mental Health at the University of Melbourne, Australia. He completed his doctorate at Deakin University in Melbourne in 2000 and has worked as a clinical psychologist in adolescent and adult public mental health settings. His research primarily focuses on psychological and pychosocial interventions in first-episode psychosis, specifically on functional recovery in first-episode psychosis, with a particular emphasis on vocational rehabilitation. Dr Killackey is also interested in evidence-based interventions in mental health and barriers to their implementation. He is a founder of the International First Episode Vocational Recovery group and was awarded the Organon Research Award in 2008 by the Australian Society for Psychiatric Research.

Pat McGorry is the director of the ORYGEN Youth Health and Research Centre, at the University of Melbourne, Australia. He has contributed significantly to research in the area of early psychosis over the past 16 years. During this time, he has played an integral role in the development of service structures and treatments specifically targeting the needs of young people with emerging or first-episode psychosis. In the past 2 years, he has published over 50 articles and chapters. Professor McGorry is the president of the International Early Psychosis Association and an executive board member of the International Society for Psychological Treatments in Schizophrenia and Related Psychosis. He is also a member of the organizing committee of the World Psychiatric Association Section on Schizophrenia, the advisory board of the University of California, Los Angeles Center for the Assessment and Prevention of Prodromal States, the editorial board of *Schizophrenia Research*, and the advisory editorial board of the *Journal of Psychiatrie Sciences Humaines Neurosciences*.

Steffen Moritz is an associate professor at the Center for Psychosocial Medicine at the University Hospital Hamburg-Eppendorf, Germany. He is an active researcher in the fields of neuropsychology and metacognition with a main focus on schizophrenia and obsessive–compulsive disorders. After receiving his diploma in psychology in 1997, he became a research assistant at the Psychiatric University Hospital of Hamburg, Germany, and obtained his PhD in 1999. Under the supervision of Professor Naber, Dr Moritz is in charge of the clinical neurocognitive unit of the hospital. Together with Dr Todd Woodward from Vancouver, Canada, he has developed a metacognitive training program for schizophrenia patients, which is now available in 23 different languages.

Ingo Schäfer is a research fellow and clinical lecturer at the Department of Psychiatry and Psychotherapy and the Center for Interdisciplinary Addiction Research at the University Medical Center Hamburg-Eppendorf, Germany. He is also an associate lecturer for public mental health at the Hamburg University of Applied Sciences. He studied medicine and public health at the Universities of Tübingen, Bordeaux, Lausanne, and Hamburg, and the Hamburg University of Applied Sciences, and received his doctoral degree from the University of Hamburg in 2002. Dr Schäfer's clinical and research interests include the treatment of patients with comorbid substance abuse and psychiatric disorders, trauma-related disorders, and treatment-resistant schizophrenia. During the past 10 years, he has been continuously involved in research on the consequences of psychological trauma in different populations and is leading various projects in that domain.

Britta Galling is a practicing psychiatrist and a researcher at the University Hospital Hamburg-Eppendorf. She studied medicine and social psychology at the universities of Hamburg, Bordeaux, Melbourne, and Montréal. Since 2003 Dr Galling has explored the subject of physician–patient communication – as a lecturer at the Institute of Medical Sociology at the University of Hamburg, and within her thesis "*Migration, Health, and Intercultural Communication.*" Beside medical anthropology and intercultural psychiatry, Dr Galling's main interest is adolescent psychiatry with a focus on psychosis. At present she is working on a project in prevention, early intervention, and integrative care in adolescent psychosis.

Liz Rietschel is a psychologist at the University Hospital Hamburg-Eppendorf, Germany. She studied psychology at the universities of Gent, Valencia, and Trier. Her special interest is the research on the treatment, prevention, and early intervention of psychosis. She gained significant experience in the subject of physician–patient communication, as she therapeutically applies individual psycho-educational approaches and cognitive behavioral treatment strategies in her work with patients at high risk for or already suffering from psychosis.

Tim Lambert is professor of psychiatry at the Concord Clinical School at the University of Sydney in Australia. He also holds an appointment as the head of the Schizophrenia Treatment and Outcomes Research unit at the Brain and Mind Research Institute in Sydney. In addition, Dr Lambert fulfills clinical duties for the Sydney Local Health Network as the director of the Centre of Excellence in Relapse Prevention in Psychosis, and at the Concord Centre for Cardiometabolic Health in Psychosis.

Philippe Conus is a professor of psychiatry and the medical director of the Service of General Psychiatry of the Department of Psychiatry, Centre Hospitalier Universitaire Vaudois in Lausanne, Switzerland, and a senior lecturer at the University of Melbourne, Australia. He completed both trainings for internal medicine and psychiatry in Lausanne. From 2000 to 2003, Dr Conus worked as a consultant psychiatrist in the Early Psychosis Prevention and Intervention Centre in Melbourne, where he developed a specialized program for early intervention in affective psychosis and a clinical research project on first-episode mania. Since returning to Switzerland, he has been heading the service of general psychiatry as well as a specialized integrated early intervention program for psychosis (Treatment and Intervention in the Early Phase of Psychosis) combining clinical and research programs. His research interests cover clinical intervention in early psychosis, the early phase of bipolar disorders, as well as neurobiological mechanisms involved in the development of schizophrenia and pharmacogenetic determinants of side effects of atypical neuroleptics.

Frauke Schultze-Lutter is a senior psychologist at the Research Department of the University Hospital of Child and Adolescent Psychiatry Bern, Germany, and the psychological-scientific head of the Bern Early Recognition and Intervention Center, a cooperation of the University Hospitals of Psychiatry as well as of Child and Adolescent Psychiatry Bern and the Soteria Bern. She studied clinical psychology in Göttingen, Germany, and received her PhD in clinical psychology at the Department of Psychology of the University of Cologne, Germany. Dr Schultze-Lutter's research focuses on the early detection of and intervention in at-risk states of severe mental disorders, particularly psychosis and bipolar disorders, with a special interest in very early subjective symptoms (ie, basic symptoms). She is the principle investigator of an epidemiological study on the prevalence of current at-risk criteria of psychosis and their relation to help-seeking, funded by the Swiss National Foundation. She was awarded the Gerd Huber Award for Research on the Prevention of Psychoses in 2010, is an elected board member of the International Early Psychosis Association, and an editorial board member of *Clinical Neuropsychiatry* and *Psychosis*.

Benno Schimmelmann is an assistant professor at the University Hospital of Child and Adolescent Psychiatry, University of Bern, where he is the chief physician and head of the research department. He studied medicine in Munich and Hamburg, Germany, and performed his child and adolescent psychiatric training at the Department of Child and Adolescent Psychiatry and Psychotherapy of the University Hospital Hamburg-Eppendorf. Dr Schimmelmann's current research interests focus on early detection and intervention in early-onset mental disorders, particularly early psychosis and bipolar disorder, and the genetics of attention-deficit/hyperactivity disorder and autism spectrum disorders. He is an associate editor of *Early Intervention in Psychiatry* and a junior editor of *European Child and Adolescent Psychiatry*.

Stephan Ruhrmann is an associate professor of psychiatry and an assistant medical director at the Department of Psychiatry and Psychotherapy of the University of Cologne, Germany, where he also heads the Cologne Early Recognition and Intervention Center and is the director of the Cologne Cognitive Neurophysiology Laboratory. He studied medicine in Heidelberg and Kiel, Germany, and performed his psychiatric training at the Department of Psychiatry and Psychotherapy of the University of Bonn, Germany. Dr Ruhrmann's current research interests focus on the prediction and prevention of psychosis. Related research activities comprise the development of multivariate prediction models and investigation of the neurophysiologic (ie, event-related potentials, eye tracking) aberrations characterizing at-risk and prepsychotic states. A further related field of his interests is the neurobiology and the prediction of negative symptoms. He was a coprincipal investigator and coordinator of the European Prediction of Psychosis Study, at present the largest prospective study in this field, and is an associate editor of *Early Intervention in Psychiatry* and an editorial board member of *Neurology, Psychiatry and Brain Research.*

Preface

It is with pride and pleasure that we have produced the third edition of the book *Current Schizophrenia*. In line with the first two editions, this publication provides valuable information and guidance for those who are involved in the care of people who have schizophrenia and their relatives. The primary intention of the book is again to provide a tool that is helpful in the treatment and care of individuals with schizophrenia and easy to use in daily clinical practice.

Many experts have devoted numerous hours to this project. Special thanks go to Dr Eóin Killackey, Professor Steffen Moritz, Associate Professor Ingo Schäfer, Professor Philippe Conus, Dr Britta Galling, Dipl Psych Liz Rietschel, Professor Tim Lambert, Dr Frauke Schultze-Lutter, Associate Professor Stephan Ruhrmann, and Professor Benno Schimmelmann, who have been directly involved in writing and/or reviewing various parts of the book. In addition, Pat McGorry has participated indirectly through his work on the Australia and New Zealand Guidelines for the Treatment of Schizophrenia.

It is exciting to see that awareness of schizophrenia has improved and continues to grow, hopefully at a rapid pace. This is important for obtaining support for research and, of course, for those who suffer from this disorder and their families. Better understanding of the disease by the society in general will help all of those affected by schizophrenia, bringing them empathy and compassion, and maybe even saving some lives. All of the contributors to this book hope that it will help with some of the issues and challenges that schizophrenia presents, and improve the quality of life of patients and their relatives. In the interest of furthering the knowledge of schizophrenia, the authors welcome any constructive criticism and comments on the contents of this book.

Dedication

This book is dedicated to Anna Joelle and Gabriele.

Chapter 1

Introduction

Martin Lambert and Dieter Naber

Advances in pharmacotherapy and psychosocial interventions continue to improve the success of managing schizophrenia. Early detection and intervention in people with, or at risk for, psychosis give patients and their families hope for a better course of illness and an improved outcome. The interdisciplinary approach, combining pharmacotherapy and psychosocial interventions, markedly increases the chance of long-lasting remission and recovery. However, a cure for schizophrenia has yet to be found. Research, particularly in the past decade, has revealed some of the biological and genetic facets of the origins of schizophrenia, and this has contributed to the better quality of treatment.

This book aims to provide a short but detailed overview of current standards of care in schizophrenia. It takes into consideration several treatment recommendations proposed in published guidelines for schizophrenia, including the guidelines by the National Institute for Health and Clinical Excellence (2009), the American Psychiatric Association (2004), the Canadian Psychiatric Association (2005), and the Royal Australian and New Zealand College of Psychiatrists (2005) [1–4]. A major problem with guidelines such as these is the difficulties encountered in translating them into daily clinical practice. Therefore, the fundamental aim of this book is to present the guidelines as clearly as possible in the context of relevant clinical treatment issues. The book does this with the help of figures that provide the clinician with algorithms and summaries of

M. Lambert and D. Naber, *Current Schizophrenia*,
DOI: 10.1007/978-1-908517-68-5_1,
© Springer Healthcare, a part of Springer Science+Business Media 2012

the most important information required for the practical treatment and theoretical understanding of schizophrenia.

The book is divided into three main chapters: current topics, organization of care, and quick reference. Chapter 2 (current topics) brings together issues of recent interest and includes sections on clinical problems and treatment of special populations. Again, Chapter 2 has been expanded considerably since this book's first publication. In addition to the pre-existing sections on first-episode psychosis, suicidality, cognitive dysfunctions, nonadherence and service disengagement, comorbid substance abuse disorders, childhood trauma, and new antipsychotics and antipsychotic formulations, this third edition includes a new section on the early detection and treatment of prodromal psychosis patients.

Chapter 3 (organization of care and treatment) provides reviews of the most important treatment recommendations in schizophrenia, including the following:

- acute and long-term treatment guidelines in first- and multiple-episode patients, including detailed pharmacological and psychosocial treatment recommendations;
- guidelines for the pharmacological and psychosocial management in special clinical situations (ie, behavioral emergencies and treatment-resistant schizophrenia);
- the management of important psychopharmacological side effects; and
- the most recommended psychosocial interventions.

Chapter 4 (quick reference) provides short overviews of the epidemiology, etiology, and the course of schizophrenia, as well as short reviews of its clinical presentation and diagnosis.

At the end of the book there is a section on resources, which includes websites that provide further information for clinicians, patients and relatives, a section on useful assessment scales, which gives an overview of the most important measurement scales in schizophrenia and, finally, further reading, which brings together the key references. To facilitate easy access, further reading is sorted alphabetically by topic.

References

1   The 2009 National Institute for Health and Clinical Excellence guideline on core interventions in the treatment and management of schizophrenia in adults in primary and secondary care (updated edition). The National Institute for Health and Clinical Excellence website. www.nice.org.uk/guidance/CG82/NICEGuidance. Accessed April 2, 2012.

2   The 2004 American Psychiatric Association practice guideline for the treatment of patients with schizophrenia. 2nd edn. www.psychiatryonline.org/content.aspx?bookid=28&sectionid=1665359#45859. Accessed April 2, 2012.

3   Canadian Psychiatric Association. Clinical practice guidelines. Treatment of schizophrenia. *Can J Psychiatry.* 2005;50(suppl 1):7S-57S.

4   Royal Australian and New Zealand College of Psychiatrists Clinical Practice Guidelines Team for the Treatment of Schizophrenia and Related Disorders. Royal Australian and New Zealand College of Psychiatrists clinical practice guidelines for the treatment of schizophrenia and related disorders. *Aust N Z J Psychiatry.* 2005;39:1-30.

Chapter 2

Current topics

Early detection and treatment of patients symptomatically at-risk for psychosis

Frauke Schultze-Lutter, Stephan Ruhrmann, Benno Schimmelmann

Over the last two decades, the treatment of psychosis has advanced substantially; yet, despite all progress, the immense individual and societal burden associated with psychosis, particularly due to schizophrenia, has largely stayed the same. Retrospective studies on the often years-long prodrome of psychotic disorders have shown that the vast majority of patients develop, among others, cognitive, perceptive, negative, and affective symptoms as well as precursors of positive symptoms and a significant loss of functioning even during the early phase of illness. Further, a long duration of untreated psychosis (DUP; time between the onset of the first frank psychotic symptom and the first adequate treatment) and a long duration of untreated illness (time between the onset of the first prodromal symptom and the first adequate treatment), have both been linked to a more negative outcome. For these reasons, an indicated prevention strategy of psychotic disorders and their negative consequences before they set in is regarded as the most promising approach to the management of these disorders.

Other than in universal preventive approaches, which utilize completely benign interventions broadly across the general population, indicated preventive approaches focus on patients with first signs of

M. Lambert and D. Naber, *Current Schizophrenia*,
DOI: 10.1007/978-1-908517-68-5_2,
© Springer Healthcare, a part of Springer Science+Business Media 2012

the emerging disorder and use specific interventions, which are not necessarily completely benign. Thus, to limit the adverse effects and cost of treating individuals who may not require treatment, a reliable and valid early detection method is necessary to select patients who are at risk of developing psychosis.

Early detection of at-risk states of psychosis

Over the last two decades, two complementary main approaches to an early detection have been developed: (1) the ultra-high risk (UHR) criteria and (2) the basic symptom criteria.

Although differences predominately occur in timing the criteria and consideration of functional decline as well as in the consideration of disorganized and negative symptoms, the UHR criteria generally involve attenuated positive symptoms (APS), brief limited intermittent psychotic symptoms (BLIPS), and/or a combination of a genetic risk factor with a recent functional deterioration (Figure 2.1). Of these criteria, APS are consistently the most frequently endorsed, and are present in about 80% of UHR patients across studies [2]. They have therefore recently been proposed for inclusion in the forthcoming 5th edition of the *Diagnostic and Statistical Manual of Mental Disorders* (DSM-V) due to be published in 2013 – and possibly in the *11th Revision of the International Classification of Diseases* projected for release in 2015 – as an attenuated psychosis syndrome (Figure 2.2) [3,4].

UHR criteria were originally designed to predict a high immediate risk of transition to psychosis within 1 year. Whilst the first studies seemed to support this assumption with 1-year transition rates of up to 50% [5–7], lower transition rates in recent studies have led to the generally accepted 1-year transition rate in UHR patients of about 20% [2]. Yet, even this lower estimate is several hundred times higher than the incidence rate in the general population of 0.035%, and studies with longer observation periods indicate a further increase in transition rates to psychosis beyond the first year to at least up to 35% [9]. More recently, interest in the longitudinal outcome of UHR patients beyond psychosis has grown. Initial studies on UHR patients undergoing diverse treatments, including antipsychotic medication, revealed remission rates

The ultrahigh risk criteria for transition to psychosis according to the Structured Interview for Psychosis-Risk Syndromes

Attenuated psychotic symptoms

Any one of the following symptoms that are qualitatively below the threshold of frank psychosis:

- **Abnormal or unusual thought content:** "magical" thinking that influences behavior and is inconsistent with subculture norms; ideas of reference and/or alien control ("Ich-Störungen"); paranoid, grandiose, somatic and/or other unusual ideas that are puzzling, preoccupying, or distressing and may affect functioning but are not held with delusional conviction
- **Abnormal suspiciousness,** ranging from slight mistrustful behavior and/or recurrent yet unfounded sense that people might be saying or thinking negative things about the person, to an anxious, unsettled state of mind with potential guarded presentation that may hinder the clinical interview
- **Perceptual abnormalities** (eg, acoustic, visual, olfactory, gustatory, tactile, somatic): persistent and puzzling perceptual distortions; recurrent unformed images, such as shadows, trails, or sounds (including hearing one's own name being called); illusions, pseudohallucinations, and/or hallucinations that are perceived as external but not yet as real and distinct from the person's thoughts (skepticism can be induced)
- **Abnormal organization of communication:** single incoherent words; temporarily going "off-track," or some loosening of association, circumstantial or tangential speech; responsive to structuring of the interviews, prompts, or questions

AND

Symptoms have begun or worsened in quality in the past year

AND

Symptoms occured at least once per week for the last month

Brief Limited intermittent psychotic symptoms

Any one of the following frank psychotic symptoms:

- **Delusions** including severe suspiciousness held with conviction that interfere with thinking and behavior
- **Hallucinations** perceived as real and distinct from the person's thoughts that interfere with thinking and behavior (skepticism cannot be induced)
- **Formal thought disorders** such as unintelligible speech or loose, irrelevant, or blocked thoughts that do not respond to structuring of the interview

AND

Symptoms have begun in the past 3 months

AND

Symptoms occur currently at least several minutes per day at least once per month

Genetic risk plus recent deterioration

At least one **first-degree relative with history of any nonaffective or affective psychosis**

OR

Schizotypal personality disorder in patient

AND

Substantial functional deterioration in the past year (defined as a drop in the Global Assessment of Functioning score of at least 30% during the last month compared to the patient's highest score in the previous 12 months)

Figure 2.1 The ultrahigh risk criteria for transition to psychosis according to the Structured Interview for Psychosis-Risk Syndromes (continues overleaf).

The ultrahigh risk criteria for transition to psychosis according to the Structured Interview for Psychosis-Risk Syndromes (continued)

General exclusion criteria

Past or present psychosis can be ruled out (ie, psychotic symptoms have never occurred for more than 1 hour per day and more than four times per week within 1 month and/or have never been disorganizing or dangerous)

AND

Symptoms are not sequelae of drug or alcohol use

AND

Symptoms are not better explained by another organic or mental disorder

Figure 2.1 The ultrahigh risk criteria for transition to psychosis according to the Structured Interview for Psychosis-Risk Syndromes (continued). Adapted from McGlashan et al [1].

Criteria of the attenuated psychosis syndrome proposed for the DSM-V

All six of the following:
- Characteristic symptoms: at least one of the following in attenuated form with intact reality testing, but of sufficient severity and/or frequency that it is not discounted or ignored:
    – delusions
    – hallucinations
    – disorganized speech
- Frequency/currency: symptoms must be present in the past month and occur at an average frequency of at least once per week in the past month
- Progression: symptoms meeting the first criterion must have begun or significantly worsened in the past year
- Distress/disability/treatment seeking: symptoms are sufficiently distressing and disabling to the patient and/or parent/guardian to lead them to seek help
- Symptoms are not better explained by any other DSM-V diagnosis, including substance-related disorder
- Clinical criteria for any DSM-V psychotic disorder have never been met

Figure 2.2 Criteria of the attenuated psychosis syndrome proposed for the DSM-V. Adapted from the American Psychiatric Association [3].

from their UHR status – but not necessarily from mental problems – of at least 50% within 1 year [11,12]. For the assessment of UHR criteria, special interview scales were developed that allow a sufficiently reliable rating when applied by trained clinicians (eg, the North-American Structured Interview for Psychosis-Risk Syndromes and the Australian Comprehensive Assessment of At-Risk Mental States) [1,13].

Whilst the information from different sources is integrated in the assessment of UHR criteria (eg, patient's report, third party's report, and interviewer's observations), the assessment of at-risk criteria according to the basic symptom concept exclusively relies on the report of the patient and, therefore, on his/her self-perception and insight; the interviewer only makes sure that the reported complaint truly meets the definition of the basic symptom in question. Basic symptoms are subtle and subjectively experienced subclinical disturbances in drive and stress tolerance that affect thinking, speech, bodily and sensory perception, motor action, and central-vegetative functions. Such symptoms can occur decades before the onset of frank psychosis. By definition, they differ from what is considered to be one's "normal" mental self and are not evoked by substance misuse or somatic illness. They remain predominately private and apparent only to the affected person and are rarely directly observable to others. Due to the emphasis on the subjective and self-experienced character, basic symptoms differ from negative symptoms, which are now predominately assessed as deficits in behavior observable to others.

Spontaneously and immediately self-recognized as mental changes, basic symptoms are also distinct from frank or more severe attenuated psychotic symptoms that are experienced by the patient as real normal thinking and feeling. Yet, although insight that something is wrong with one's mental processes is present, some experiences might be so new and strange that they remain nearly inexplicable. Hence, a detailed description of these experiences usually requires help in the form of guided questioning by trained interviewers. The ability to experience basic symptoms with insight and to cope with them, however, often attenuates with progressive illness (ie, with emerging psychotic symptoms and more severe APS), but is restored upon remission.

There are two criteria used to assess basic symptoms: COgnitive-PERceptive basic symptoms (COPER; Figure 2.3) and COGnitive DISturbances (COGDIS; Figure 2.4) [14–17]. Despite their partial overlap in symptoms, the two criteria slightly differ in their predictive accuracy: whilst COPER performs better in ruling out subsequent psychosis (ie, has a lower rate of false-negative predictions and a higher sensitivity), COGDIS performs better in ruling in subsequent psychosis (ie, has a lower rate of false-positive predictions and a higher specificity). Naturalistic long-term follow-up studies reported transition rates to first-episode psychosis (FEP) within an average period of 10 years (minimum 5 years; no antipsychotic treatment before onset of psychosis) and within 4 years (various treatments including antipsychotic treatment before the onset of psychosis), respectively, of 65% and 38% for COPER and 79% and 39% for COGDIS [18]. Across studies, the average 1-year transition rate of both basic symptom criteria is about 20% [14].

The basic symptom criteria: COGDIS

Any two of the following nine basic symptoms with at least weekly occurrence within the previous 3 months:

- **Thought interference:** an intrusion of completely insignificant thoughts that are not related to the intended thought and hinder concentration and thinking without resulting in a loss of the train of thoughts
- **Thought pressure:** a self-reported "chaos" of thoughts; a great number of random, different thoughts or images enter the mind and disappear again in quick sequences without the ability to suppress or guide them; the successive thoughts are completely unrelated to each other or to the intended content of the patient's thinking
- **Thought blockages:** a subjective blocking of thought that can also be experienced as a sudden emptiness of thoughts, interruption of thoughts, fading (slipping) of thoughts, or losing the thread of thoughts. The original topic might subsequently be recalled or completely lost
- **Disturbance of receptive speech:** a disturbance in the immediate comprehension of simple words and sentences, either read or heard, that can result in giving up reading or avoiding conversations; it resembles "normal" problems with second languages, when a word is recognized as familiar but one cannot recall it, or its meaning is delayed
- **Disturbance of expressive speech:** self-experienced problems in producing appropriate words, sometimes also experienced as a reduction in active vocabulary; a self-recognition of verbal fluency, precision, and availability of language being slowed down
- **Disturbance of abstract thinking:** deficits in the comprehension of any kind of abstract, figurative, or symbolic phrases or contents as well as phenomena of concretism; an exceptional basic symptom that can either be self-reported or observed and rated when tested (eg, by asking to explain sayings or idioms)
- **Inability to divide attention** between simultaneous nondemanding tasks that each draw primarily upon a different sense that would not usually require a switching of attention; generally at least one demand is performed on a (semi-)automatic level and does not require full attention (eg, a patient may not be able to listen and pay attention to an oral presentation and take down notes at the same time; or cannot prepare a sandwich and talk to a family member at once)
- **Captivation of attention by details of the visual field** that catch and hold the look and attention; an ordinary visual stimulus or part of it stands out strikingly, appears almost isolated from the rest of the environment and is emphasized so that this single aspect of the environment catches and captures the attention completely; might also be described as a "fixation of perception" or "spell-bounding"
- **Unstable ideas of reference** with immediate insight into the pathological, "weird" nature of the feeling of reference (ie, a vague feeling that random events or comments and actions by others were related to oneself, while instantly knowing that this is impossible or at least most improbable). Other than in ideas of reference, the feeling of reference is not considered as reality-based, and no cognitive processes like reasoning or weighing pros and cons are involved before overcoming the idea (reality testing is completely intact)

Figure 2.3 The basic symptom criteria: COGDIS. Adapted from Schultze-Lutter et al [14].

The basic symptom criteria: COPER

Any one of the following ten basic symptoms WITH at least weekly occurrence within the prior three months AND first occurrence at least twelve months ago:

- **Thought interference** (see Figure 2.3)
- **Thought perseveration:** an obsessive-like repetition of banal thoughts or images of no emotional significance that can be related to all possible trivial past events; these "memories" are so unimportant and lacking in emotion that, even in the patient's evaluation, they do not justify the excessive mental occupation given to them
- **Thought pressure** (see Figure 2.3)
- **Thought blockages** (see Figure 2.3)
- **Disturbance of receptive speech** (see Figure 2.3)
- **Decreased ability to discriminate between ideas and perception, fantasy and true memories:** a disturbance in the ability to surely distinguish internal, mentally generated events from external, perceived or experienced events, leading to a difficulty in locating the source of the experience/memory (not rated if the patient questions certain perceptions or does not fully trust himself anymore)
- **Unstable ideas of reference** (see Figure 2.3)
- **Derealization:** a change in how one relates emotionally to the environment with two potential forms:
  1. An alienation from the visual world (ie, how one sees the world). The environment appears unreal, changed and strange in a way that is often hard to describe. Here the individual feels estranged from the world and the usual emotional ties to the surroundings no longer exist or have become considerably weaker; a feeling of being disconnected from the environment.
  2. An increased emotional affinity for the environment. The environment, or certain isolated aspects of it, are exceptionally emotional impressive; often accompanied by rather positive or euphoric feelings
- **Visual or acoustic perception disturbances** with immediate complete insight. Unlike hallucinations or schizotypal perceptual distortions, perceptual basic symptoms are not regarded as real but are immediately recognized as a sensory or subjective problem. The knowledge that the misperception (eg, a wrong coloring, distorted shape or changed sound quality/intensity), has no counterpart in the real world is immediate and unquestioned

Figure 2.4 The basic symptom criteria: COPER. Adapted from Schultze-Lutter et al [14].

Studies combining UHR criteria, particularly APS, and basic symptom criteria, particularly COGDIS, indicate that the combined presence of APS and COGDIS signals the highest short-term risk of transition (within 1 to 2 years) compared to the presence of either criterion alone [10]. Further, in a recent meta-analysis of studies employing different at-risk criteria, the transition rate appeared to be influenced by the particular at-risk criteria that were employed, with higher rates reported in studies employing the basic symptom approach as compared to studies employing the UHR approach [19].

In conclusion, the 1-year incidence rates of psychosis in at-risk patients (predominately adult or mixed adult and adolescent samples) are generally several hundred times higher than the 0.035% rate in the general population. However, the still high proportion of seeming false-positives, at least within shorter follow-up periods, has fostered ethical concerns about unnecessary preventive measures and stimulated a search for additional predictors. Further, about 18% of patients with FEP have the onset of the full-blown disorder before the age of 18 years, and an even more significant proportion of patients has the onset of the prodrome in childhood and adolescence [20]. Thus, it still remains to show that at-risk criteria are unaffected by potential developmental peculiarities and are also valid to a similar degree in these young age groups.

Other disturbances in at-risk states of psychosis

One indisputable general finding resulted from the studies searching for additional predictors to increase the predictive ability of existing at-risk criteria: irrespective of a future development of psychosis, people presenting at mental health services with at-risk criteria suffer from a large variety of other psychopathological symptoms or even mental disorders. The most common symptoms and disorders include depressive disorders and social phobia, functional deficits (including deficits in stress coping strategies), and deficits in social cognition, and affect regulation and meta-cognition, such as negative beliefs about an individual's own ability to control events. Further, among others, at-risk persons exhibit neurocognitive deficits (particularly in verbal fluency and memory, working memory, and processing speed), electrophysiological aberrations indicative of a gating deficit, local reductions of gray matter (particularly in cingular structures), and deficits in functional MRI indicative of a hypofunction of the prefrontal cortex, as well as aberrations in PET and MRS studies pointing toward disturbances in serotonergic and dopaminergic neurotransmission, and an increased level of anandamide in the cerebrospinal fluid. In addition, they report a reduced quality of life that is similarly impaired to that of FEP patients.

In light of the impressive and still growing evidence of deficits in this group of help-seeking patients, above and beyond their potential risk of psychosis, their clinical status clearly meets DSM-IV-TR criteria of a mental disorder that is "conceptualized as a clinically significant behavioral or psychological syndrome or pattern that occurs in an individual and that is associated with present distress (…) or disability (ie, impairment in one or more important areas of functioning) or with a significantly increased risk of suffering death, pain, disability, or an important loss of freedom" [21]. Therefore, these patients should be considered as "ill" and in need of treatment.

Early intervention in at-risk states of psychosis

Despite the need for treatment for present symptoms and problems, early intervention studies have mainly focused on the prevention of future psychotic symptoms above the threshold for full-blown psychosis. Though the number of early intervention studies is still limited and study samples had often been small, encouraging results have already been reported from pharmacological and psychotherapeutic trials. And a recent review of five randomized controlled studies (two based on medication, two on psychological or psychosocial treatment, and one on a neuroprotective fatty acid treatment) concluded that receiving any focused treatment was associated with a lower risk of developing psychosis as compared to no treatment or treatment as usual, indicating a relative risk of 0.36 (95% CI, 0.22–0.59) in the treatment group at the time of treatment cessation [22]. In most studies, however, this "preventive" effect was not stable after treatment cessation, indicating a delay rather than a prevention of psychosis.

Initial early intervention studies in UHR and related samples, each comprising only approximately 60 participants, were modeled on treatments for full-blown psychosis and mainly applied low-dose medication with antipsychotic drugs (risperidone and olanzapine) with or without additional psychotherapy or cognitive–behavioral psychotherapy, not excluding use of antipsychotics [23–25]. A phase-specific treatment approach was followed in the German Research Network on Schizophrenia, in which two larger early intervention trials were conducted, each including approximately 120 patients. One study explored the effects of cognitive–behavioral therapy in at-risk patients identified by COPER and/or an adapted UHR genetic risk criterion [26]; the other studied the effects of low-dose amilsulpride in at-risk patients reporting APS or BLIPS [27]. The studies differed in the length of the treatment period (between 6 months and 2 years) and terminated according to study protocols irrespective of the clinical state.

However, studies are frequently evaluated under the presumption that an intervention can only be regarded as successful when its effects remain after treatment cessation. Yet to do so, a successful intervention with long-term effect would have to override the impact of a highly complex interplay of genetic, epigenetic, neurodevelopmental, and psychosocial factors that start at conception and determine the risk of, and progression to, psychosis. In somatic disorders with longstanding risk conditions, long-term rather than short-term intervention is therefore a common strategy (eg, in the prevention of stroke). As implied by the concept of indicated prevention, however, this would certainly require treatment strategies with a very favorable cost–benefit ratio for at-risk individuals. Thus, current concepts of an effective prevention in terms of time-limited interventions should be reconsidered.

A promising new road to the prevention of psychosis, which is not modeled on treatments of frank psychosis but a unique opportunity in the early states, is based on a recent neuroprotective intervention study. In this randomized controlled study of a 3-month high-dose treatment with omega-3 fatty acids in a sample of 81 UHR patients [28], the effectiveness in preventing transition and improving current symptoms indicated that it may indeed be possible to develop benign interventions particularly for the at-risk state, independent of their effectiveness in manifest psychosis, that, furthermore, have lasting effect after treatment cessation. Though a long-term effect of a well-tolerated substance would be the most desired and would present a therapeutic breakthrough, these first results still have to be confirmed and extended, particularly with regard to truly long-term effects spanning years. Moreover, it will be necessary to investigate whether such preventive treatment is also efficient in adults past the main years of brain development. Also, should larger replication studies reveal that a short-term intervention is not as sufficient as the first study has suggested, long-term tolerability of high doses of omega-3 fatty acids will have to be studied.

In summary, it is most important to intensify basic research efforts in these early stages and to develop new special early intervention approaches from these findings. Furthermore, recent observations indicate that at least the temporal variance of risk estimation by UHR criteria is broader than originally expected. Therefore, improved enrichment strategies or clinical staging algorithms that allow a more individualized risk classification or stratification have to be developed to increase the homogeneity of individual risk levels in study samples; this might prove a necessary precondition for conclusive risk-adapted prevention trials. However, after preventive intervention strategies have proven their efficacy in studies on at-risk patients seeking help in specialized services, the next challenge will be to prove the effectiveness of an early intervention at epidemiological level (ie, with regard to all subjects at increased risk of developing psychosis and not only the subsample of those seeking help early).

To conclude, although the first one and a half decades of early detection and intervention research in psychosis have already produced encouraging results, much remains to be done before evidence-based, detailed intervention guidelines can be developed and implemented into clinical settings. Until then, the rather vaguely defined guidelines formulated in 2005 by the International Early Psychosis Association (IEPA) writing group (Figure 2.5), which are due to be updated, will have to serve as a general framework to the clinical handling of people exhibiting potential at-risk symptoms of psychosis.

First-episode psychosis
Eóin Killackey

FEP presents a great opportunity to provide quality interventions, positively engage the patient in treatment of the psychosis, and minimize the secondary disability that can stem from psychosis. The 2005 IEPA guidelines on the interventions for FEP are summarized in this chapter.

Two important dimensions of interventions for FEP are the timing of the intervention (and therefore DUP) and the quality of the intervention (the sustained provision of comprehensive phase-specific treatment).

Treatment guidelines of the International Early Psychosis Association writing group

If young people with an at-risk mental state are actively seeking help for the distress and disability associated with their symptoms, they need to be:

- Engaged and assessed
- Offered regular monitoring of mental state and support
- Offered specific treatment for other syndromes, such as depression, anxiety, or substance misuse, and assistance with problem areas such as interpersonal, vocational, and family stress, if present
- Provided with psychoeducation and encouraged to develop coping skills for subthreshold psychotic symptoms
- Offered family education and support
- Provided information in a flexible, careful, and clear way about risks for mental disorders as well as about existing syndromes

Such care can be carried out in a low stigma environment, such as home, primary care, or a youth-friendly office-based setting

Antipsychotic medications are not usually indicated unless the person meets criteria for a DSM-IV/ICD-10 psychotic disorder. Exceptions should be considered when rapid deterioration is occurring; severe suicidal risk is present, and treatment of any depression has proved ineffective; or aggression or hostility are increasing and pose a risk to others. If antipsychotics are considered, ideally, atypical medications should be used in low doses and considered as a "therapeutic trial" for a limited period. If there is benefit and resolution of symptoms after 6 weeks, the medication may be continued with the patient's consent for a further 6 months to 2 years, following explanation of risks and benefits. After this period, a gradual attempt to withdraw the medication should be made if the patient agrees and there has been a good recovery. If the patient has not responded to one atypical antipsychotic, another may be tried if the above indications still exist

If young people with an at-risk mental state are not seeking help, then regular contact with family members or friends may be an appropriate strategy

The evidence of the effectiveness of treatments aimed specifically at reducing the risk of transition to psychosis (eg, cognitive and family therapy, antipsychotic medication, or experimental neuroprotective drug strategies) remains preliminary. More data are required and the risk–benefit ratio of various interventions needs to be determined

Figure 2.5 Treatment guidelines of the International Early Psychosis Association writing group. Adapted from the International Early Psychosis Association Writing Group [29].

Although this topic is beyond the scope of this book, identification and treatment of people at risk of psychosis have resulted in the reduction of DUP to zero.

Often, as a result of both the nature of onset of psychosis and resource issues in mental health care systems, there are prolonged delays in initiating effective treatment for FEP. Although there was previously some debate, prolonged DUP is now known to be independently associated with poorer response and outcome. The clinical staging model being applied to mental illnesses suggests that identification of patients in the earliest phases of psychotic disorders allows for more optimal treatment, and is likely to reduce the burden of disease while it is active. Any improvements in long-term outcome should be seen as a bonus, rather than as a prerequisite for improving clinical standards during early illness.

FEP tends to be more responsive to treatment than subsequent episodes; later phases of illness tend to be less stable and may evolve over time, making definitive diagnosis more difficult. The umbrella term "psychosis" accommodates this syndromal flux and comorbidity, and allows treatment to be commenced for all prominent syndromes before a definitive diagnosis, such as schizophrenia, can be or has to be applied. Thus, whether core schizophrenia can be diagnosed is not crucial for effective treatment in FEP. A notable example is that cannabis use is common in FEP and can cause confusion and delay in treating the psychotic episode. Significant cannabis use appears to be a risk factor for the onset of schizophrenia, as well as an aggravating factor for the subsequent course. It is crucially important, therefore, that there is no disconnect between the management of the substance abuse and the mental disorder; rather, a unified approach is called for. Recommendations for treatment of FEP are listed in Figure 2.6.

Recommendations for treatment of first-episode psychosis

- Strategies to improve the treatment of first-episode psychosis include better mental health literacy, more informed primary care, and greater responsiveness of public and private psychiatry to possible cases. Community-wide education systems should be developed to improve understanding of how psychotic disorders emerge in a previously healthy person and how to seek and obtain effective advice, treatment, and support
- A high index of suspicion and a low threshold for expert assessment should be set
- Entry and retention within specialist mental health services is often based on a reactive, crisis-oriented model, in which patients must reach a threshold of behavioral disturbance, risk, disability, or chronicity before they are retained. This model is a poor use of resources and creates unnecessary trauma, demoralization, and therapeutic nihilism in patients, families, and clinicians. Instead, services should aim for proactive retention of patients throughout the first 3–5 years of illness, combining developmental (youth) and phase-specific perspectives
- Initial treatment should be provided in an outpatient or home setting, if possible. Such an approach can minimize the trauma, disruption, and anxiety of the patient and family, who are usually poorly informed about mental illness and have fears and prejudices about in-patient psychiatric care. In-patient care is required if there is a significant risk of self-harm or aggression, if the level of support in the community is insufficient, or if the crisis is too great for the family to manage, even with home-based support

Figure 2.6 Recommendations for treatment of first-episode psychosis (continues overleaf).

Recommendations for treatment of first-episode psychosis (continued)

- In-patient care should be provided in the least restrictive environment. Optimal in-patient units should be streamed by phase of illness and developmental stage, be relatively small in size, and be staffed adequately, so that one-to-one nursing of highly distressed, suicidal or agitated young people is possible, without locking sections of the unit or secluding the patient, unless this is absolutely necessary. The use of traditional psychiatric intensive care, a pragmatic intervention that lacks a solid evidence base, is especially traumatic for these patients. Where streaming is not possible, a special section may be created in a general acute unit for young recent-onset patients
- Pharmacological treatments should be introduced with great care in medication-naïve patients to do the least harm while aiming for the maximum benefit. Appropriate strategies include graded introduction, with careful explanation, of low-dose antipsychotic medication, plus antimanic or antidepressant medication, where indicated. Skilled nursing care, a safe and supportive environment, and regular and liberal doses of benzodiazepines are essential to relieve distress, insomnia, and behavioral disturbances secondary to psychosis, while antipsychotic medication takes effect
- The first-line use of atypical antipsychotic medication is recommended on the basis of better tolerability and reduced risk of tardive dyskinesia. In the longer term, the risk–benefit ratio may change for some patients (eg, if weight gain or sexual side effects associated with the atypical agents develop). Typical antipsychotic medications may then be one of the options considered
- Initial assessment should include a baseline computed tomography scan, neurocognitive screen, neurologic examination for movement disorder, electrocardiogram, body mass index, and a fasting serum glucose level
- Psychosocial interventions, especially cognitive–behavior therapy (CBT), are an important component of early treatment, providing a humane basis for continuing care, preventing and resolving secondary consequences of the illness, and promoting recovery. CBT may also be helpful for comorbid substance use, mood and anxiety disorders, and improving treatment adherence
- Families and, whenever possible and appropriate, other members of the patient's social network, should be supported actively and educated progressively about the nature of the problem, the treatment, and the expected outcomes. If there are frequent relapses or slow early recovery, a more intensive and prolonged supportive intervention for families is required
- If recovery is slow and remission does not occur despite sustained adherence to two antipsychotic medications (at least one of which is an atypical medication) for 6 weeks each, early use of clozapine and intensive CBT should be considered seriously
- Early use of clozapine should also be considered if suicide risk is prominent or persistent

Figure 2.6 Recommendations for treatment of first-episode psychosis (continued). Adapted from McGorry et al [30].

As stated, FEP is a prime opportunity for intervention. The earlier and more appropriately this intervention begins, the better. An optimal and sustained intervention at this point has the greatest possibility of reducing the secondary disability wrought by psychosis. In addition, it increases the probability of better quality-of-life outcomes for the patient. To achieve these objectives, a goal-oriented framework focused on recovery is required, rather than a mindset that concentrates on chronicity and disability. Good practice in this area is to stay abreast of the development of pharmaceutical and psychological therapies targeted at FEP, incorporate evidence-based guidelines developed around FEP into clinical practice, and convey optimism and hope to those experiencing FEP and to their families and friends.

Cognitive dysfunctions in schizophrenia
Steffen Moritz

Many patients with schizophrenia display severe neurocognitive dysfunction in a wide variety of domains, most notable memory and executive functioning. These dysfunctions are in most cases present at the first exacerbation but, unlike Kraepelin's initial concept of "dementia praecox" at the end of the nineteenth century, do not necessarily progress during the course of the illness, beyond age-related decrement. Although neurocognitive deficits are not obligatory for diagnosis, the necessity for their identification and treatment in schizophrenia is increasingly acknowledged.

In the past decade, a large body of empirical evidence has been accumulated showing that cognitive disturbances are important determinants of functional outcome variables such as social relationships and work status. For example, in a meta-analysis, it was demonstrated that memory dysfunction is a particularly strong predictor of functional outcome in schizophrenia [31]. In addition, there is increasing recognition of the impact of neuropsychological dysfunction on a number of treatment-related variables, such as insight and coping skills.

Neurocognitive dysfunction may also exert a negative impact on compliance with medication. For example, several psychotropic agents, especially benzodiazepines and anticholinergic medications, with the latter often being prescribed to attenuate the side effect of conventional neuroleptics, are known to have potential adverse effects on neurocognition in some patients. When such side effects remain unnoticed, drug discontinuation may occur, especially if the patient considers that the adverse side effects outweigh the benefits of drug treatment.

Evaluation of negative medication effects is also essential, given that many patients are already cognitively impaired before treatment, potentially compromising the outcome of psychotherapeutic or psychoeducational treatment. Memory problems and dysfunctions in abstract logical thinking may severely limit the outcome of insight-based psychotherapeutic interventions. A compromised capacity to store information, as evidenced by many psychiatric patients, as well as older patients with or without mental illness, may also lead to forgetfulness about taking medication and the purpose and contents of psychotherapy, with forgetting about the latter being a further risk factor for noncompliance. Recently, we found that approximately one third of patients with schizophrenia do not take their medication as prescribed because of prospective memory problems.

Once neurocognitive problems have been detected, there are a number of strategies that can be used to deal with such dysfunctions in psychiatric patients. With regard to memory problems, clinicians should repeat essential information regularly, check from time to time that patients are indeed grasping the core aspects of therapy, give the most essential information in written form (especially on medication and dosage, but also for cognitive–behavioral intervention and stress management) and, when appropriate, involve relatives in the session so that they can remind patients in their own homes. To illustrate, the effects of psychoeducation are usually more effective when relatives are involved. Patients with decreased sustained attention benefit from more frequent but shorter therapeutic sessions. In addition, there is evidence that cognitive remediation programs are effective for at least some patients. The administration of second-generation antipsychotics may ameliorate some neurocognitive symptoms (possibly via the improvement of negative symptoms), or at least may not aggravate neurocognitive dysfunctions. However, in view of conflicting new evidence on the neurocognitive effects of atypical antipsychotics, a seemingly closed chapter has been reopened.

Clinicians may want to evaluate whether medications that are potentially harmful to memory, such as benzodiazepines and anticholinergic agents, are still necessary or could at least be diminished in dosage. In any case, the presence of memory and other neurocognitive problems should not be disregarded as a minor problem or lesser evil given their possible impact on compliance with medication, insight, treatment, and functional outcome. In addition, cognitive dysfunctions may cause increased stress at work or school, because many jobs necessitate intact selective attention, vigilance, and memory. To compensate for neurocognitive problems, the impaired patient must devote more effort to a task than individuals whose cognitive functioning is normal. However, this causes stress, a major risk factor for renewed exacerbation of psychiatric symptoms according to the widely accepted vulnerability–stress model of psychiatric illness. This creates a vicious circle when job demands are not suited to the patient's cognitive abilities.

Cognitive biases and metacognitive training in schizophrenia

In addition to neurocognitive impairment, cognitive biases (or cognitive distortions) are being increasingly investigated. This line of research encompasses a wide variety of response styles and cognitive distortions. Prominent biases are jumping to conclusions (eg, hasty decision making), deficits in theory of mind (eg, failure to empathize with others and to deduce motifs), a bias against disconfirmatory evidence, overconfidence in errors, negative self-schemata, and monocausal attributional styles. There is evidence that these styles are related to the emergence and maintenance of psychotic symptoms, especially delusions, in concert with other factors. Importantly, these cognitive distortions seem to precede psychotic breakdown and the patient is not fully aware of them (ie, many patients lack metacognitive insight into these problems). Hence, a training program, entitled metacognitive training (MCT), has been developed (Figure 2.7). Its eight modules aim to raise the patient's awareness of these distortions and to prompt the patient to critically reflect on, complement, and change his or her current repertoire of problem solving. Thus, its main purpose is to change the "cognitive infrastructure" of delusional ideation. As psychosis is rarely an instantaneous incident, changing the appraisal of one's cognitions and social environment may act prophylactically on psychotic symptoms. The modules are administered in the framework of a group intervention program. Several studies

Summary of each metacognitive training module

Module	Target domain	Description of core exercises
1. Attribution: blaming and taking credit	Self-serving bias versus depressive attributional style	Different causes of positive and negative events must be contemplated. For example, "a friend was talking behind my back"; dominant interpretation: "friend is not trustworthy" (blaming others); alternatives: "I have done something bad" (blaming self), "she is preparing a surprise party for my birthday" (circumstances). Explanations that take into account various causes are preferred to monocausal explanations. The negative consequences of self-serving attribution are repeatedly highlighted
2. Jumping to conclusions, I	Jumping to conclusions; liberal acceptance; bias against disconfirmatory evidence	Motifs contributing to hasty decision making are discussed and its disadvantages are stressed. Fragmented pictures are shown that eventually display objects. Premature decisions often lead to errors, emphasizing the benefits of cautious data gathering. In the second part, ambiguous pictures are displayed. Here, a quick survey leads to the omission of details demonstrating that first impressions may often reveal only half the truth
3. Changing beliefs	Bias against disconfirmatory evidence	Cartoon sequences are shown in backward order, which increasingly disambiguate a complex scenario. After each new picture, patients are asked to (re-)rate the plausibility of four interpretations. Although the initially most likely interpretation prevails in some pictures in the course of the exercises, patients are "led up the garden path" on others. Thus, patients learn to withhold strong judgments until sufficient evidence has been collected, and encouraged to maintain an open attitude toward counter-arguments and alternative views
4. Empathy, I	Theory of mind, first order	Facial expression and other cues are discussed for their relevance to social reasoning. Pictures of human faces are presented in the exercises. The group should guess what the depicted character(s) may feel. The correct solution often violates a first intuition, demonstrating that relying on facial expression alone can be misleading. In the second part, cartoon strips are shown that either must be completed or brought into the correct order. Participants are shown that social inferences should involve multiple cues

Figure 2.7 Summary of each metacognitive training module (continues opposite).

Summary of each metacognitive training module (continued)

Module	Target domain	Description of core exercises
5. Memory	Overconfidence in errors	Factors that foster or impair memory acquisition are discussed first, and examples for common false memories are presented. Then, complex scenes (eg, beach) are displayed with two typical elements removed (eg, towel, ball). Owing to logical inference, gist-based recollection and liberal acceptance, many patients falsely recognize these lure items in a later recognition trial. The constructive rather than passive nature of memory is thus brought to the participants' attention. Patients are taught to differentiate between false and correct memories by means of the vividness heuristic
6. Empathy, II	Theory of mind, second order; need for closure	Different aspects guiding theory of mind (eg, language) are discussed with respect to both their heuristic value and fallibility for social decision making. Then, cartoon sequences are presented, and the perspective of one of the protagonists must be considered, which involves discounting knowledge available to the observer but not available to the protagonist. For the majority of sequences, no definitive solutions can be inferred, which is unsatisfactory for patients with an enhanced need for closure
7. Jumping to conclusions, II	Jumping to conclusions/liberal acceptance	As in module I, the disadvantages of quick decision making are outlined with regard to events related and unrelated to psychosis. In the exercises, paintings are displayed, for which the correct title must be deduced from four response options. On superficial inspection, many pictures tempt false responses
8. Mood and self-esteem	Mood and self-esteem	First, depressive symptoms, causes, and treatment options are discussed. Then, typical depressive cognitive patterns in response to common events are presented (eg, overgeneralization, selective abstraction), and the group is asked to come up with more constructive and positive ones. At the end, some strategies are conveyed to help patients to transform negative self-schemata and elevate their mood

Figure 2.7 Summary of each metacognitive training module (continued). Reproduced with permission from Moritz et al [32].

assert the feasibility of this approach as well as its efficacy. MCT can be downloaded cost-free in 23 languages from www.uke.de/mkt. A number of self-conducted as well as independent investigations have affirmed the feasibility, safety, and efficacy of this approach as an add-on treatment to standard intervention. Since 2008, an individualized version called MCT+ has also been available from www.uke.de/mkt_plus.

Suicidality in schizophrenia

Martin Lambert

Suicide is the most frequent cause of death in patients with schizophrenia. Estimates of completed suicides by patients with schizophrenia range from 4% to 13%, similar to the range seen in affective disorders [33,34]. This is approximately four times higher than in the period before deinstitutionalization (1913–1960) [35], which has been interpreted as suggesting that the suicide rate has risen markedly since the onset of deinstitutionalization. However, recent re-evaluation of previous studies has concluded that the suicide rate is in fact lower, at approximately 5%, and that this rate is 7–10 times higher than in the general population [36]. Approximately 40–50% of individuals with schizophrenia either consider or attempt suicide [37–39]. In the prodromal and/or untreated psychotic phase before first treatment contact, 5–15% of patients with schizophrenia attempt suicide [40]. The high proportion of suicide attempts that result in death can be explained by the high autoaggression of the attempts.

In general, it can be assumed that psychoreactive and social consequences of schizophrenia are the primary causes of suicidal behavior, especially when accompanied by a depressive affect. There are various risk factors for suicide attempts and completed suicide in schizophrenia; some of them are similar to those in the general population, and others are specific to the disorder itself (Figure 2.8). Most patients fulfill several of these risk factors concurrently, so there are certain risk constellations that are especially predictive for suicidal behavior. For example, a high risk was found for single, unemployed males with severe forms of schizophrenia, previous suicide attempt(s), and concurrent depressive episodes

Risk factors related to suicidal behavior

- Previous suicide attempts and actual suicidal ideation and/or plans
- Recent depressive episode and/or lifetime major depressive episode(s), especially in combination with hopelessness
- Long duration of untreated psychosis; possibly also long duration of untreated illness
- Severe forms of the disorder; paranoid subtype with suspiciousness and agitation in the absence of negative symptoms, impulsivity
- Comorbidity, such as substance use disorder or obsessive–compulsive disorder
- Poor adherence to treatment or service disengagement
- Socially isolated single males; lack of support and/or occupation; homelessness
- Relatively higher premorbid functioning before onset of psychosis (eg, higher education); relatively higher cognitive functioning including intelligence and self-expectations; greater insight into illness, but also problem-solving deficits
- First 10 years of illness; frequent short hospitalizations in past year; first 6 months after discharge from hospital
- Repeated unsuccessful antipsychotic treatment attempts with side effects (especially akathisia)

Figure 2.8 Risk factors related to suicidal behavior.

and/or substance abuse disorders. In summary, the main factors to be taken into account when assessing risk of suicidal behavior in patients with schizophrenia are previous suicide attempts, recent or past affective symptoms or syndromes, recent suicidal thoughts, threats or suicidal behavior, poor adherence to treatment, fears of the impact of illness on a patient's life, and substance abuse.

Prevention of suicidal behavior and suicide is likely to result from ongoing community and professional education, early detection, and early intervention, as well as active treatment of the underlying causes. The latter mainly includes treatment of affective symptoms and syndromes, improving adherence to treatment, use of medication that may have special antisuicidal effects, and ongoing special vigilance when patients have a number of risk factors, especially if the impact of the disease on the patient's functional level and quality of life is significant.

The optimal management of suicidality in schizophrenia involves early detection and regular assessment of suicidal ideation, immediate and effective interventions to ensure safety, selection of psychosocial interventions based on the patient's needs, and pharmacotherapy directed primarily at psychotic and depressive symptoms (Figure 2.9). Pharmacological treatment for suicidality should consist of additional supportive medication to alleviate the emotional pressures. This alleviation can be achieved with sedative or anxiolytic drugs, such as benzodiazepines, or antipsychotic

Recommendations for the management and treatment of suicidal behavior in schizophrenia

Strive for early detection and regular assessment	• The risk of suicide and suicidal behavior in schizophrenia is significant and matches that of affective disorders. The clinician needs to be alert to subtle hints of suicidality, particularly during high-risk periods. Suicide in schizophrenia is often not impulsive, as it is commonly believed
Assess risk factors and risk constellations	• Assessment of risk factors and risk constellations is vital in the management of suicidal behavior in schizophrenia. This includes, for example, initial assessment of duration and severity of suicide intent, previous suicidal ideation or attempt, mediating factors (both risk and protective factors [see Figure 2.8]), phase and severity of psychotic (eg, command hallucinations) and associated symptoms (eg, agitation), degree of subjective distress, level of affective disturbance, access to lethal means, supervision and support available, potential for treatment nonadherence or service disengagement, and patient's initial response to clinical interventions proposed. Check that patient has not made recent attempt that might require immediate treatment
Ensure immediate safety	• Ensure patient's immediate safety by providing constant supervision and removal of any potential means to self-harm until an appropriate intervention has been decided upon
Decide on appropriate management plan	• Determine who will be the primary clinician involved and facilitate the establishment of a therapeutic alliance between the patient and that clinician throughout the high-risk period • Liaise with patients' other treating clinicians, check immediately available interventions, and consult with senior clinical staff if high suicide risk is determined. Liaise with carers regarding recent and past history of factors that might indicate increased suicide risk. Determine degree of supervision needed to minimize likelihood of a suicide attempt, balancing degree of suicide intent, willingness to comply, variability of mental state, and reliability of the least restrictive options available. Decide on necessary treatments, and negotiate options with the patient (eg, hospitalization)
Initiate management plan	• Supervision: Provide an adequate level of supervision by staff or carers with clear instructions about risk, degree of monitoring, frequency of clinical reviews needed, and responses required if a deterioration is observed (eg, who and how to consult if problems arise) • Safety: Remove access to means of self-harm (eg, razors, knives, cords, guns, medications, and poisons). Limit exposure to immediate stressors and, if necessary, provide containment within a safe setting (eg, hospital, with clear instructions to carers about limitations on patients' freedom) • Personal contact and counseling: Provide initial counseling and treatment while establishing rapport, understanding, and trust; explore cognitions that influence level of suicidality; encourage an understanding that suicide ideation is a transient although painful phenomenon related to illness; instill hope in recovery through treatment; and finally negotiate a suicide contract • Initiate treatment: Reduce associated distress due to psychosis or suicide ideation with anxiolytics (eg, benzodiazepines) and/or antipsychotics. Attempt to influence psychosocial factors that might reduce suicidality (eg, practical assistance with homelessness, access to social milieu)

Figure 2.9 Recommendations for the management and treatment of suicidal behavior in schizophrenia (continues opposite).

Provide optimal pharmacologic treatment	• Medication(s) to treat suicidality in schizophrenia should fulfill the following criteria: (1) eliminate positive symptoms, (2) enhance quality of life through improved depressive symptoms, anxiety, and social functioning, (3) be free of extrapyramidal symptoms, and (4) decrease substance use. Clozapine has been shown to have a substantial effect on both attempted and completed suicide. It should be considered in patients showing significant suicidal behavior, though other atypical antipsychotics may be useful in patients for whom clozapine is either contraindicated or otherwise undesirable
Review management	• Regularly review and negotiate the above interventions with the patient, carers, and other clinicians involved. Ensure clear lines of clinical accountability and decision making

Figure 2.9 Recommendations for the management and treatment of suicidal behavior in schizophrenia (continued). Adapted from Power et al [41].

drugs or, particularly in the long term, clozapine. Patients for whom clozapine is appropriate are those who have made serious suicide attempts on other medications, and are likely to follow the generally accepted guidelines for taking clozapine. If patients refuse clozapine or are unable to tolerate it, there is no evidence to assist in making the choice among the other antipsychotic drugs. Overall, a second-generation antipsychotic drug would be superior to a first-generation agent, based on the greater tolerability, enhanced effect on depression, and possibly lower risk of noncompliance. The pharmacotherapy of the underlying disorder should also be re-evaluated with respect to efficacy and tolerability.

Nonadherence and service disengagement in schizophrenia

Britta Galling, Liz Rietschel, Martin Lambert

Introduction

Poor adherence to medication as well as to treatment in general (referred to as treatment engagement or service disengagement) is one of the main treatment problems in schizophrenia. Rates of medication nonadherence within the first 2 years after hospital discharge are approximately 50–75% [42], and 20–40% for service disengagement within the first 18 months [43,44]. However, current reviews on medication nonadherence suggest that these rates are probably even higher [42]. A variety of risk factors have been identified, which increase the risk of medication nonadherence and poor treatment engagement. The prediction of nonadherent behavior by these risk factors is complicated, as they can change and interfere with each other over time. Consequences of medication nonadherence and service disengagement are manifold and lead to a poor course of illness and worse overall prognosis. A variety of clinical interventions have been described for an improvement in treatment engagement and specifically in medication adherence. However, an integrated approach gives the highest chance for long-lasting improved adherence in individual patients. This chapter provides a brief yet detailed overview of various aspects that play a role in medication nonadherence and treatment disengagement.

Definition

Adherence is defined as the extent to which a patient complies with the physician recommendations. Unlike compliance, adherence focuses on following the course of action that was mutually agreed upon by the patient, the physician and, when appropriate, the caregivers.

An essential prerequisite for adherence is that the patient has been adequately informed, understands different therapeutic treatment options, and has chosen an appropriate treatment in accordance with the physician. The participation of the patient in the process of the decision-making (ie, shared decision-making) is already well established in other medical domains. It is based on the general societal trend for more autonomy and self-determination, better information availability on the internet and other media, and the advancement of patients' rights. However, patients' rights to shared decision-making involve difficulties in daily practice for several reasons, which can be especially significant in case of psychiatric disorders. First, patient involvement lessens the aspect of the paternal and directive relationship between a patient and a physician. Second, it requires good communication skills on part of the physician, which are usually not sufficiently taken into account during their professional education. Third, the decision-making ability in patients, especially in those suffering of psychosis, is often challenged and can be limited, at least temporarily.

At present, shared decision-making is the best-defined concept for facilitating patient involvement in antipsychotic management for those suffering from schizophrenia.

Models of adherence

There are two overlapping categories of adherence to therapy:

1. Medication adherence, which refers to the antipsychotic medication, other psychotropic drugs (eg, mood stabilizers), somatic medication (eg, antihypertensive therapy), or the overall drug treatment. Studies have shown that nonadherent behavior usually affects the overall drug treatment and is not limited to medication for a particular disorder. The stage of adherence is expressed by the percentage of medication that was not taken as prescribed:
   - full adherence: <20% of the medication missed;
   - partial adherence: 20–80% of the medication missed; and
   - full nonadherence: >80% of the medication missed.
   Furthermore, a special category of nonadherence includes the so-called "medication refusers." These patients, due to persistent nonadherence, have never received antipsychotic or other drug treatment in the required duration and/or amount. An epidemiological study assessing adherence in 605 first-episode patients found that 18.8% of the patients belonged to that group [43].
2. Adherence to the entire treatment regimen (treatment engagement), where nonadherence is defined as the overall therapy dropout rate. In the majority of cases, patients drop out after multiple attempts to continue with treatment. Clinical studies show that 20–40% of the patients abort overall therapy in the first 12–18 months after hospital discharge [43–45].

Examination methods

There is no gold standard for the measurement of adherence, and the determination of individual adherence is based on an assessment of a patient's current behavior. The following methods can be employed in adherence assessment:

- a patient's own declaration (assessed by an interview and/or questionnaires);
- assessment by a physician or pharmacist (assessed by an interview and/or questionnaires);
- reports by family members or caregivers;
- assessment of medication collection/purchase;
- observation of intake (eg, hospital ward, therapeutic flat share);
- pill counting;
- calculation of medication availability over time;
- Medication Event Monitoring System® (electronic monitoring of extraction of capsules/pills from a container); and
- in vitro diagnosis (ie, blood sample analysis).

In 161 adherence studies conducted from 1971 to 2006, Velligan et al found that 124 studies (77%) were based solely on subjective statements (eg, by patients or clinicians; Figure 2.10) [46]. However, the measurement methods have been reported to differ considerably with regards to their

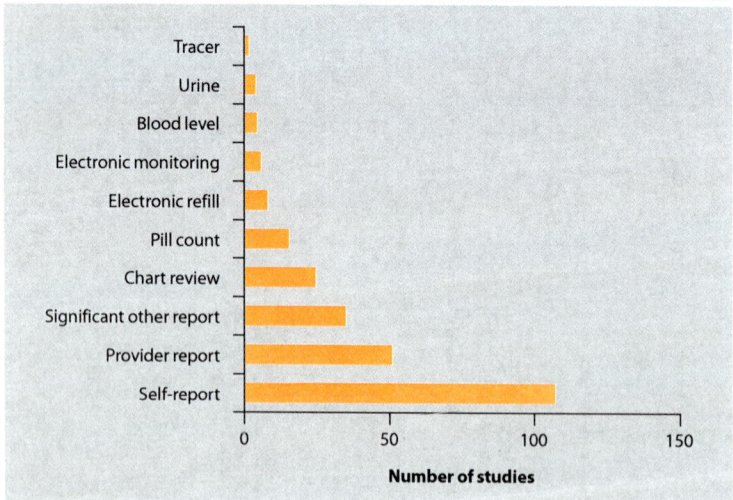

Figure 2.10 Method of adherence assessment in 161 studies from 1971 to 2006. Reproduced with permission from Velligan et al [46].

validity. Velligan et al showed clear differences in adherence rates 3 months after inpatient discharge depending on the measurement used (subjective patient statements: 55%; counting pills: 40%; blood level: 23%) [46]. These results suggest that the extent of nonadherence in patients with schizophrenia is larger than previously believed.

Frequency

Studies on the frequency of partial or complete antipsychotic treatment adherence show large methodological differences, especially with regards to the measurement of adherence, duration of the studies, and study populations. An important limitation of almost all studies is that, in most cases, unrepresentative (nonepidemiological) patient cohorts were analyzed. Real high-risk nonadherence patients were often not included and not analyzed, as they mostly do not take part in "informed consent" studies. The methodological heterogeneity causes a significant variance in the determined nonadherence rates, which range from 20% to 89%. If only the studies with reliable methodology are included, the 1-year nonadherence rates are approximately 40–50%, and up to 75% of patients are partially or wholly nonadherent within 2 years after discharge from a hospital [46]. The following conclusions can be made regarding the frequency of nonadherent behavior:

- The studies with fewer selectively chosen patient populations have higher rates of partial or complete nonadherence. This insight must be taken into account in interpreting the majority of adherence studies.
- In nonselected cohorts there is, as mentioned earlier, a subgroup of patients known as medication refusers, who, when not treated under monitoring conditions, do not accept antipsychotic medication, at least for some period of time.
- The rates of partial or complete nonadherence rise with increasing duration of treatment.

Causes and risk factors

Knowledge of risk factors of partial or complete nonadherence is vital for planning an effective treatment regimen that is simple to adhere to. Different authors have proposed different systematization of risk factors, including categories based on patient-associated factors, relationship-related aspects (ie, family and social support), and factors associated with the care system (Figure 2.11).

In order to fully understand the risk factors for nonadherence, it is important to remember that they are not static, but rather can be positively influenced by treatment. It is not necessarily the risk status at admittance that determines the adherence, but whether and how the risk factors evolve during treatment. For example, a patient's familiarity with the disease influences adherence; however, it is less important whether a patient is familiar with the disease when admitted than it is how effectively he is informed about the disease during the course of treatment. The same is true for other factors, including the presence of a comorbid addictive disorder, attitude toward treatment, supportive therapeutic alliance, and an adequate medication supply system.

Consequences

It is well known that partial or complete nonadherence (to medication or to the entire treatment) is an important factor in the course of the disease and the prognosis. Accordingly, nonadherent behavior is directly or indirectly associated with the following consequences:

- increased recidivism (psychotic or comorbid) leading to higher doses of antipsychotic medication, increased polypharmacy, and more adverse events;
- partial response or nonresponse to treatment and therapy resistance;
- increased inpatient treatment with higher costs;
- increased emergencies;
- chronicity of schizophrenic and comorbid symptoms;
- a decreased level of functioning and quality of life; and
- increased suicide attempts.

It is important to understand that these consequences can be caused even by partial nonadherence.

Therapeutic measures for improved adherence

The complexity of the problem of nonadherence becomes clear in clinical experience: some patients enjoy the benefits of treatment and willingly

Risk factors for partial and complete nonadherence	
Patient-associated factors	• Poor insight into disease and treatment
	• Negative attitude or subjective response toward medication
	• Shorter illness duration (first-episode psychosis)
	• Comorbidity, especially persistent substance use disorder
	• Cognitive impairment
	• Fear of side effects and addiction
	• Fear of stigma
	• Past nonadherence
	• Demographic factors such as lower age and male gender
	• Social factors such as living alone and unemployment
Other factors (including relationship-related aspects and factors associated with the care system)	• Insufficient therapeutic alliance
	• Insufficient family and social support
	• Deficient care systems, including long latency time and lack of finances to afford appropriate medication
	• Complex route of medication administration
	• Severity of adverse events

Figure 2.11 Risk factors for partial and complete nonadherence. Based on data from Lacro et al [47] and Goff et al [48].

take medication, others do not like and do not take medication, yet others dislike some aspects of treatment but take medication as prescribed. There is no single intervention that can solve the problem of nonadherence. Instead there are a number of possible interventions, which should be adapted to the patient's individual condition, and which need to be further adjusted over the course of treatment.

The first step: physician–patient relationship and participative decision making
Physician–patient relationship
An attitude to sickness in general and to any disease in particular is strongly influenced by the societal factors, varies significantly by culture, and evolves with time. A disease and its symptoms are thus a phenomena, which could be considered and evaluated differently from variable viewpoints of doctors, patients, and the society. This is especially true for psychiatric diseases such as schizophrenia. Hence it is important to take into account that in the treatment of psychosis, the patients' concepts of disease, corresponding treatment designs, and expectations of treatment are strongly influenced by the experiences and attitudes of the patient. An important prerequisite for improving adherence is to address

and understand these perceptions and attitudes and to take them into account while planning treatment. A decisive factor in this process is the quality of communication and interaction between the person providing the treatment and the patient. An effective physician–patient interaction provides the patient with necessary information and an opportunity to contribute to the therapeutic decision making, which improves the process of diagnosis, understanding of and coping with the disease, and therefore the adherence to therapy and the efficiency of treatment.

Communication in the physician–patient relationship

The physician–patient interaction is strongly characterized by an asymmetry, which resonates in all communication processes. The doctor is active, performs the usual professional role, and knows the rules and procedures of the clinical setting. He or she possesses expert knowledge and uses technical terminology. The patient, on the contrary, is more passive, and due to the illness, which is usually a dramatic event for the patient, may be unsettled, anxious, and stressed. He or she is torn out of their normal daily life, is dependent on specialists, has only layperson knowledge, and may be unfamiliar with the clinical setting. In patients with psychosis, such an asymmetry in the physician–patient relationship can have a significant influence on adherence. The goal for a physician must therefore be to build a relationship with a patient that is as symmetrical as possible, where the patient is informed about the disease and therapy decisions can be made together. This process of "shared decision-making" should be the first step to increasing the patient's willingness to adhere to treatment.

Shared decision-making

The term shared decision-making was defined in 1982 by the President's Commission for the Study of Ethical Problems in Medication and Biomedical and Behavioural Research [49]. However, in a 2006 review comparing different studies on shared decision-making, Makoul et al found that the definition of this term had remained largely unchanged [50].

The general and most important idea of shared decision-making is that the physician should attempt to inform the patient as well as potential caretakers about the disease and therapy options. In doing so, the physician imparts his or her knowledge advantage to the patient, and after this stage the therapy decisions should be made together.

According to Makoul et al physicians have variable understanding of shared decision-making, and assumptions vary widely regarding how to proceed in working with the patient to select appropriate therapy (Figure 2.12) [50]. Some doctors assume that it is their responsibility to convince the patient to take the most appropriate medication; others think that their role is to recommend a medication, and to leave the final decision of whether or not to agree to it to the patient. This discrepancy hinders the ability to compare the research on the effectiveness, and of other factors involved in shared decision-making.

At the start of therapy and during the course of the disease, individual factors that influence short- and long-term risks for nonadherence and therapy dropout should be raised frequently by physicians and assessed in collaboration with the patient.

Further therapeutic measures for improving adherence

There is no single measure that can solve the problem of nonadherence. A number of interventions can be implemented based on the patient's individual conditions. Most patients profit from multimodal therapeutic approaches, which can change over the course of treatment. Risk factors can fluctuate over a period of time and influence one another. Accordingly, it is important to regularly check therapy adherence and adjust the interventions.

The following therapeutic measures can be used to help improve adherence:

- **Cognitive–behavioral therapy:** The first step in the behavioral therapy involves identification of cognitive and behavioral patterns that negatively influence the patient's wellbeing. During the course of therapy, the patient learns certain techniques that can be utilized to alter these patterns. For example, negative attitudes toward medication use can be discussed and cognitively restructured, and new strategies for regular therapy participation can be worked out. The educational part of the behavioral therapy

Essential elements of shared decision-making

1. Define/explain the problem

Factors that seem problematic to the physician may not be important to the patient, and vice versa; a patient may be concerned with some factors that may be incidental in the physician's perspective. Therefore, it is not enough to simply inform the patient of the diagnosis. The physician must understand and address the patient's perception of the disease and any concerns that may arise and interfere with treatment

2. Present options to solve the problem

Any discussion between the physician and the patient about potential solutions to the problems and challenges faced by the patient is indispensable. The physician's role is mainly to provide education and further information on the origins and the course of disease and different approaches to therapy

3. Consideration of advantages and disadvantages of treatment

Considering all the advantages and disadvantages of a specific treatment strategy is an important step in physician–patient communication, especially when the physician's and patient's opinions differ widely. The patient's personal values and preferences should be considered and taken into account during the decision-making process. For example, if the patient has an impression that he will not benefit from the therapy or may be harmed by side effects, extra time should be dedicated to discuss these attitudes

4. Discussion of patient's abilities and self-efficacy

Patients with psychosis frequently have difficulties with therapy adherence because of forgetfulness and lack of structure and organization in their lives. Furthermore, patients with psychiatric diseases tend to lack self-confidence, which is associated with lower expectations in one's ability to deal with the disease. Consequently, some patients may think that they are unable to change their current condition and confine themselves to a passive role during the therapy process. Physicians should discuss this aspect and ensure that the patients understand that they can influence the treatment and the prognosis by adopting a more proactive approach

5. Physician's knowledge and recommendations

In this step, the physician should list all possible treatment strategies and identify the best approach. The physician should not seem patronizing, but rather consider himself a consultant. The patient should not feel like he is being pushed toward a certain treatment

6. Ensuring patient's understanding

The next step is to ensure that the patient understands what is being said. Therefore, complex terms should be either avoided or precisely explained. The physician also has to be certain that he fully understands all the patient's expectations, fears, and concerns

7. Making or delaying decisions

The final step involves a decision on the treatment strategy and a mutual agreement by the physician and patient on that approach. One cannot assume that this will be possible at the end of the initial consultation. Additional time and consultations may be necessary depending on the form and degree of the disease, psychological strain, and patient's opposition. The patient should not feel pressured to make a decision immediately. If desired, additional appointments should be made to further discuss various treatment strategies and concerns

Figure 2.12 Essential elements of shared decision-making. Adapted from Makoul et al [50].

(both family and individual education) includes information about the basis of the disease and available treatment options. Such education can reduce the recidivism rate due to noncompliance by approximately 20% [51].

- **Adherence therapy (compliance therapy)** is a short-term intervention (usually with 4–6 sessions), based on motivational conversation with a patient. The effectiveness of this intervention has been clinically proven: patients that have participated in this therapy had a five-time higher chance of adhering to treatment.

- **Cognitive–motivational addiction therapy** is useful for patients with a comorbid addiction disorder. This therapy is used to motivate the patient to end substance abuse and can be offered both in group and individual therapy settings.

- **Assertive community treatment:** In this form of therapy patients are, if necessary, treated at home. Patients are also given an emergency number, which they can call to receive immediate help and support in case of a crisis. This form of therapy is especially recommended for ambulatory patients, who rarely have appointments in the clinical setting and regularly cease using their medication.

- **Person-to-person or family-to-family assistance:** Experienced and informed patients are increasingly given an opportunity to aid other patients. The credibility of such patients is very high as they themselves have experienced the disease and have learned to live with it. The same applies to informed family members, who can pass on their knowledge to other families. Both strategies can improve medication adherence of affected individuals.

- **Destigmatizing the disease:** People with psychiatric diseases are often stigmatized by society. The symptoms of schizophrenia, especially, can sometimes cause the behavior of affected people to breach many of the societal norms, which can lead to extreme stigmatization. Therefore, patients usually have to deal not only with the symptoms but also with the stigma, which can cause such a degree of shame and suffering that it is known as the "second disease." Not only can this limit the patient's quality of life but it can also have a great influence on the treatment and course of the disease. An open conversation on the subject of stigmatization within the doctor–patient interaction is therefore indispensable.

- **Dialogue and medicinal compliance:** Physicians need to address negative convictions that patients may have regarding their treatment, which can affect adherence. Potential topics for discussion involve likely assumptions regarding medication efficacy, potential for addiction, and undesirable side effects.

- **Technical support for medicinal compliance:** Patients with repeated nonadherence can profit from measures that simplify the administration of medication. For example, a switch from multiple daily doses to a once-a-day dose or depot medication may improve compliance. If applicable, continuous supervision of medication administration (eg, Medication Event Monitoring System™ or a nursing service) can provide necessary support, at least until the autonomous adherence is assured. In addition, it has been shown that depot medications can and should be used preventively in first-episode patients or patients with nonadherence risk factors. Every appointment should include a short screening for treatment adherence, and the patient's attitude toward medication should be assessed routinely.

Co-occurring substance abuse in schizophrenia

Martin Lambert

Co-occurring substance use disorders, often termed "dual diagnosis" or "comorbidity," are a serious and common issue among patients with schizophrenia, and frequently remain under-recognized and poorly addressed. Up to 90% of people with schizophrenia smoke cigarettes [52–54], and 40–60% use other substances [55]. Comorbid substance abuse (excluding tobacco smoking) appears to be more prevalent (up to 75%) among young people with FEP [46], as well as among those who are homeless or have come to the attention of the criminal justice system. The most frequently abused substances are cannabis, alcohol, and psychostimulants, mirroring patterns of use evident within the general population, although abuse of more than one substance is relatively common (20–40%) [56,57]. Most patients start using before the onset of psychosis (with regular cigarette use usually starting first), which most probably reflects the typical temporal order of onset of both disorders.

A number of hypotheses have been proposed to explain the high rate of co-occurring substance use among people with psychosis, including the following:

- psychosis increases risk for substance use;
- substance abuse increases risk for psychosis; and
- common factors increase risk for both disorders.

The "self-medication" hypothesis proposes that individuals with psychosis are more prone to substance abuse because they selectively abuse particular substances in order to "treat" specific symptoms of their psychotic illness. Despite the intrinsic appeal of this model, supporting evidence is limited, and factors associated with substance abuse in the general community also apply to those with psychosis (eg, cost, availability, use for intoxication and relaxation, peer group use, and acceptance). Nevertheless, people with psychosis do consistently report abusing substances to relieve feelings of dysphoria, anxiety, and boredom, and it is likely that some patients continue to abuse substances to help cope with a range of psychosocial problems (eg, family conflict, trauma, financial problems, lack of vocational opportunities, and social anxiety).

The hypothesis that substance abuse is a risk factor for psychosis has received support from a number of recent longitudinal cohort and population-based studies. Regular cannabis use appears to be associated with an approximately twofold increase in the relative risk of developing schizophrenia or other psychosis outcomes. However, although cannabis use (particularly adolescent-onset and heavy use) is a risk factor for later psychosis, the incidence of schizophrenia does not appear to be increasing despite elevated rates of cannabis use in the general community. This suggests that the relationship between cannabis use and psychosis is particularly complex, and further studies examining the interaction of genotype, developmental processes, and cannabinoid exposure are required. However, a recent population-based study in positively selected people (without psychosis risk factors) and long-term follow-up showed that cannabis use was linked to the development of psychosis and resistance to treatment in case of ongoing cannabis use [58].

An alternative hypothesis for the high rate of co-occurring substance abuse disorders among individuals with psychosis is the possibility that common underlying biological, personality, or environmental factors increase vulnerability for both disorders. For example, both disorders are associated with dysfunction within the brain's reward system, as well as frontal executive deficits, whereas certain personality traits (eg, sensation seeking, impulsivity, and negative affect) have been implicated in the etiology of co-occurring psychosis and substance use disorders. Certain personality traits (eg, antisocial personality disorder) as well as environmental experiences also increase risk for both disorders.

Cigarette smoking is associated with considerable morbidity and mortality among people with schizophrenia, yet interventions are not routinely offered to this population despite evidence for their effectiveness. Smoking also places a substantial financial burden on such individuals, who spend a large proportion of their weekly income on cigarettes.

Abuse of other substances has a significant impact on both treatment course and outcome, and many patients do poorly in standard treatment settings. Indeed, co-occurring substance use disorders are associated with lower rates of remission, frequent use of health care services and increased rates of relapse and hospitalization, blood-borne virus infections (eg, human immunodeficiency virus), suicide, violent behavior, incarceration, and early death. In addition, persistent substance abuse affects medication adherence, service engagement, health care costs, and housing stability, and substantially increases the burden on patients, their families, and the health care system. Although this often leads to clinicians feeling pessimistic toward this population, many individuals with FEP achieve remission and/or a reduction in the severity of substance abuse after entry to treatment, and a significant reduction in substance abuse is likely to be associated with improved clinical outcomes.

It is essential that all patients with psychosis are assessed for co-occurring substance use, given the high rate of substance use within this population and the associated negative outcomes (Figure 2.13).

Recommendations for the management and treatment of substance use disorder in schizophrenia

Assessment	• Screen all patients for substance use and other psychiatric disorders (eg, social phobia) • Determine severity of use and associated risk-taking behaviors (eg, injecting practices, "unsafe sex") • Exclude organic illness or physical complications of substance use • Seek collateral history: families or close supports should be involved where possible

Treatment principles	• First engage patient, adopting a nonjudgmental attitude
	• Educate patient:
	  – Give general advice about harmful effects of substance use
	  – Advise about safe and responsible levels of substance use
	  – Make individual links between substance use and patient's problems (eg, cannabis use and worsening paranoia)
	  – Inform patient about safer practices (eg, using clean needles, not injecting alone, practicing "safe sex")
	• Treat psychotic illness and monitor patient for potential side effects
	• Help patient establish advantages and disadvantages of current use, and motivate patient for change
	• Evaluate need for concurrent substance-use medications (eg, methadone, acamprosate)
	• Refer patient to relevant clinical and community services, as appropriate
	• Devise relapse prevention strategies that address both psychosis and substance use
	• Identify triggers for relapse (eg, meeting other drug users, being paid, family conflict) and explore alternative coping strategies

General interventions	• Explore reasons for substance use, including relationship to psychiatric symptoms, antipsychotic treatment, and feelings of social isolation • Address patient's motives and degree of commitment toward treatment of both their psychotic illness and substance use • Adopt concrete problem-solving approach with patient, where appropriate • Set tasks that are simple and readily achievable (eg, keeping a diary of substance use or psychotic symptoms; regularly taking medication; keeping appointments) • Focus on specific skills to deal with high-risk situations, and consider use of role play (eg, learning how to say "no" to a dealer or drug-using friends) • Suggest alternatives to substance use for coping with stressful situations (eg, exercise, contacting a support person) • Treat comorbid anxiety with behavioral techniques (eg, breathing exercises, progressive muscular relaxation) • Remain supportive and emphasize any gains made • Encourage participation in alternative activities and contact with non-substance-using peer group (discuss available resources with local community health center or mental health service)
Motivational enhancement techniques	• Motivational interviewing is a useful therapeutic approach, based on a model conceptualizing stages through which behavioral change occurs. It emphasizes the role of both ambivalence and relapse within the process of change. This therapeutic approach aims to match appropriate treatment options with the patient's motivational level, based on the patient's current stage within the cycle

Figure 2.13 Recommendations for the management and treatment of substance use disorder in schizophrenia. Adapted from Meister et al [59,60].

The assessment should include a detailed history of the type, amount, pattern, and circumstances of substance use, negative consequences associated with use (including the impact on mental and physical health, and social and occupational functioning), the degree of physiological dependence, the interaction between psychosis and substance use, relevant risk issues (eg, accidental or deliberate overdose and aggressive behavior when intoxicated), reasons for use, previous attempts to control use and past treatment, and motivation/readiness to change substance use. Assessment is most accurate if the clinician establishes a collaborative therapeutic alliance, using an empathic nonjudgmental approach. Biomedical investigations (eg, γ-glutamyl transpeptidase, urine drug screen) and collateral information should also be sought, because patients may minimize their level of substance use. It is important to assess for any level of use, because people with schizophrenia are often more sensitive to the effects of psychoactive substances and experience greater adverse effects than would typically be expected.

Psychosis in the context of co-occurring substance use presents clinicians with a particularly difficult diagnostic challenge, especially as many psychoactive substances can induce psychotic symptoms during periods of intoxication or withdrawal. That said, psychosis can also occur with prolonged abuse, and there is growing evidence that substance-induced psychotic episodes occur more frequently among individuals with substance use disorders. Although substance-induced psychotic symptoms are typically transitory in nature, generally lasting less than a week in most cases, there is a small but growing amount of literature to suggest that, in a minority of chronic users, psychotic symptoms can last substantially longer than a month (especially among those with underlying schizoid or schizotypal traits). Nevertheless, the priority of initial assessment should be to identify treatment-relevant syndromes (such as the triad of psychosis, substance abuse, and depression), and to start appropriate treatment. Indeed, those with substance-induced psychosis should not be excluded from treatment, especially as there is evidence to suggest that they are a particularly high-risk group for later transition. In this regard, the interaction between substance abuse and psychotic symptoms should be monitored longitudinally to ensure accuracy of the initial diagnosis.

It is important to acknowledge that many clinicians feel overwhelmed or not sufficiently skilled to manage patients with co-occurring disorders. Many are often pessimistic regarding outcomes and believe that substantial time and effort are required for little return. It is therefore not uncommon for clinicians to want limited involvement with such patients, and to try to refer them elsewhere. However, the reality is that few physicians have had specialized training in managing co-occurring disorders, and practitioners need to acknowledge that substance abuse is a common concomitant of a psychotic illness. It should be borne in mind that appropriate interventions have been shown to be beneficial, and clinicians need to remain optimistic with realistic long-term expectations.

Comprehensive treatment planning involves discussing the assessment with the patient (and key support/carer if the patient consents), providing education about the link between psychosis and substance abuse outcomes, identifying clear treatment goals, and discussing potential pharmacological and psychosocial interventions. The approach should be integrated, such that both the psychosis and the substance abuse are addressed simultaneously in a comprehensive treatment package. Effective pharmacological treatment of the psychotic illness with antipsychotic agents is critical, because improved medication adherence increases the effectiveness of adjunctive psychosocial interventions. In this regard, patients should be offered simplified medication regimens, as well as clear information about potential interactions between their prescribed medication and abused substances. Those who are consistently nonadherent may benefit from switching to a longer-acting depot antipsychotic, although limited research has been conducted to examine the effectiveness of this approach. Benzodiazepines should be used with caution because of their interaction with alcohol and other depressants, as well as their potential for abuse. Limited pharmacological trials for substance abuse have been conducted among patients with schizophrenia, but most addiction treatments appear to be safe and effective in combination with antipsychotics. Nicotine replacement therapies and bupropion have both been successfully and safely used in patients with schizophrenia.

Assertive outreach with intensive case management has been found to improve engagement and retention, as well as treatment outcomes, in those with co-occurring disorders; however, few such programs exist. Nevertheless, ensuring that the patient's immediate needs are addressed, as well as offering practical assistance with everyday tasks, enhances engagement and increases motivation for treatment. Life-long abstinence may be a particularly difficult goal to achieve for this population, and it is more useful to adopt a harm reduction framework focused on reducing the harm associated with the substance abuse and its consequences. In general, psychosocial interventions for substance abuse need to be modified for people with schizophrenia (eg, adopting a concrete problem-solving approach or the use of role play), given the negative symptoms, cognitive difficulties, and poor self-efficacy associated with this disorder. Motivational interviewing remains an important component of treatment, in terms of identifying the pros and cons of continuing or ceasing substance use, and accepting treatment, addressing ambivalence, building self-efficacy, identifying and implementing relevant strategies for change, encouraging new skills, and rehearsing relapse prevention strategies (for both the psychosis and the substance abuse). It is important that "lapses" are not viewed as failures, but should rather be discussed early in treatment as being something that is to be expected and viewed as an opportunity to refine the patient's set of coping strategies.

Lack of vocational opportunities, homelessness, and contact with drug-abusing peers are obvious drivers of continued substance abuse, and these should be addressed early in treatment. Vocational and educational goals are also important motivators for change, and relevant support agencies should be included in treatment planning to ensure that relevant opportunities are considered. Links to alternative social networks and support groups are also essential. Finally, families play a particularly important role in supporting and monitoring treatment, as well as building self-efficacy and self-esteem, and should be involved early in treatment planning, with the patient's consent. Carers may need additional support themselves, because family conflict is common when patients have co-occurring disorders.

Childhood trauma in schizophrenia

Ingo Schäfer and Philippe Conus

Trauma and its consequences have long been a neglected issue in patients with schizophrenia and other psychotic disorders. However, over the past decade, interest in this topic has markedly increased. The existing evidence consistently shows a high prevalence of early trauma, especially childhood sexual abuse (CSA) and childhood physical abuse (CPA), in the lives of people with psychosis. In a recent critical review of 20 carefully selected studies on patients with psychotic disorders, 42% of the female patients reported CSA and 35% reported CPA. In male patients, these figures were 28% and 38%, respectively. At least one form of abuse (CSA or CPA) was found in 50% of the patients, irrespective of gender [61]. A slightly lower prevalence of CSA and/or CPA has been reported in studies focusing on patients with bipolar disorder, but this is likely to be due in part to the dearth of studies exclusively exploring these adverse experiences in bipolar patients.

Population-based studies suggest that childhood trauma may be a causal factor for psychosis. In almost all existing studies, a history of trauma was related to psychotic symptoms during either adolescence or adulthood. For example, in a prospective study of 4045 individuals aged 18–64 years drawn from the Netherlands Mental Health Survey and Incidence study (NEMESIS), participants who had experienced emotional, physical, or sexual abuse before the age of 16 were more likely to develop positive psychotic symptoms according to several different definitions during a 3-year follow-up period, after adjusting for a wide range of potential confounding factors (adjusted odds ratio 7.3) [62].

Research into the consequences of early trauma suggests that both psychological and neurobiological factors may contribute to the development of schizophrenia and other disorders. At the psychological level, the focus has been on cognitive factors and their interplay with emotions. Neurobiological theories include alterations of the hypothalamic–pituitary–adrenal axis and an altered function of the dopaminergic system. Although some of these mechanisms have been linked to a range of mental health problems, others (eg, information processing abnormalities) might represent distinct processes specifically associated with schizophrenia and other psychotic disorders.

Psychotic patients with a history of childhood trauma have a more severe clinical profile across a variety of measures compared with those without these experiences. They have an earlier onset of the illness, a higher number of hospitalizations and a more severe clinical course. Patients with childhood trauma are more likely to have been revictimized later in life, have more current or lifetime substance abuse, and suffer from more lifetime episodes of major depression. Victims of abuse also have higher levels of current depression and anxiety, and report more dissociative symptoms than patients without these experiences. One of the most prevalent consequences of childhood abuse is posttraumatic stress disorder (PTSD). In clinical samples, the disorder is in most cases related to childhood abuse, and in a smaller group of patients to experiences later in life. Whereas about 3–5% of individuals in the general population fulfill a current diagnosis of PTSD [63], the prevalence of the disorder in samples of patients with schizophrenia is 17–46% [64,65]. Rates of current PTSD in individuals with bipolar disorder range from 11% to 24% [66,67].

In a study of patients with schizophrenia in vocational training, victims of childhood abuse had a poorer level of participation, were less able to sustain intimacy, and were more prone to emotional instability. Finally, abused patients have frequently been found to report more suicidal ideation and suicide attempts. Although similar findings with regard to the consequences of early trauma have been reported independent of psychiatric diagnosis, more specific differences have also been reported concerning the type and content of psychotic symptoms. In patients diagnosed with schizophrenia, those who suffered CSA or CPA have repeatedly been found to have more "positive symptoms" (eg, hallucinations, ideas of reference, and thought insertion) and fewer "negative symptoms" than those without a history of abuse. Although findings about the interrelationship of childhood trauma and delusions, thought disorder, and "negative symptoms" remain inconsistent, the link between childhood trauma and hallucinations has repeatedly been replicated and seems to exist across diagnostic boundaries including schizophrenia spectrum disorders, affective psychosis, personality disorders, and dissociative disorders, and also in the general population. Finally, associations can be found between childhood trauma and the actual content of psychotic symptoms; for example, schizophrenia patients with a history of childhood abuse tend to hear more malevolent voices with hallucination themes such as threat, guilt, and humiliation.

Given the strikingly high number of patients with a history of trauma and the obvious clinical problems related to this issue, recommendations have been published to design trauma-sensitive services for people with severe mental illness. They call for a more systematic assessment of trauma history, better staff training, and modification of standard services to recognize particular safety, control and boundary issues that such patients face. With regard to assessment, research suggests that instruments for identification of childhood trauma and PTSD developed for the general population are also appropriate for use among people with psychosis. Some useful observations are summarized in the following box.

Discussing previous trauma with patients who have schizophrenia
- It is important to ask patients with schizophrenia about a possible exposure to trauma:
  - Without asking, only 10–30% of trauma histories are identified [68].
  - Although trauma is very rarely a part of clinical assessment (because of other priorities for assessment, fear of destabilizing patients, doubt about veracity of reported trauma, fear of blaming families), 85% of patients who have lived through such events are relieved when they are offered an opportunity to talk about them [68].
- When trauma is discussed with a patient:
  - It is often a progressive process: it is not necessary to gather all details at once and patents need time to gradually expose what they went through.
  - Clinicians need to be available and to positively reinforce the efforts that patients make to talk about such issues.
  - It is also important to evaluate the risk for victimization, recurrence of trauma, and suicide.

Trauma-specific treatments aim to directly address the effects of abuse. Although, no sound evidence is available for differential pharmacological approaches, several psychotherapy treatments have proved effective in patients with psychosis who have experienced childhood trauma. Patients with early and complex trauma may benefit from integrated treatment programs with an emphasis on psychoeducation, stabilization, and the development of safe coping skills. Other approaches focus on PTSD. Several case studies and open trials reported that exposure-based treatments of PTSD can be used safely and effectively in patients with schizophrenia [69,70]. More recently, a randomized controlled trial of a group-based cognitive–behavioral intervention for PTSD, with an emphasis on cognitive restructuring rather than exposure therapy, has yielded promising results in patients with severe mental illness [71]. Independent of the strategy chosen, trauma treatments for patients with schizophrenia should take place within the context of a comprehensive and integrated service, where all aspects of the disorder can be addressed in a coherent fashion, combining case management, medication, and psychotherapy of the various comorbidities that may occur. Clearly, more research is needed to further develop and evaluate treatment approaches appropriate for this vulnerable population and to integrate them into routine practice.

New antipsychotics and antipsychotic formulations
Tim Lambert

In patients with schizophrenia, antipsychotics are the cornerstone of therapy for the management of an acute episode of psychosis and for prevention of relapse. They provide the bedrock upon which psychosocial treatments can be applied in order to achieve remission. Due to their lower risk of extrapyramidal adverse effects and their (variable and arguably modest) beneficial effects on the negative, affective, and cognitive symptoms of schizophrenia, the so-called atypical or second-generation antipsychotics (SGAs) are often utilized in preference to the older, conventional first-generation antipsychotics (FGAs). However, despite the oral SGAs having a preferable risk–benefit ratio, rates of persistence on these medications, dimensional improvements, and general social integration differ extensively.

The complex nature of the disease and the fact that responsiveness to any single agent is largely idiosyncratic, suggests that psychiatrists should have a broad palette of agents at their disposal in order to attempt to individualize treatment. That the rates of adherence are only marginally better with the latest medications compared to the FGAs, suggests that any individualized treatment plan also needs to consider ways of dealing with nonadherence, and this may require considering new forms of delivery of the required agent such as rapidly disintegrating tablets, sublingual preparations, and injectable short- and long-acting formulations. In the years to come, newer delivery methods such as patches, aerosols, implants, and gas-forced subcutaneous injections will extend our ability to administer agents to patients who are unable to maintain their adherence.

This chapter considers new antipsychotics that are reaching the clinic, as well as new formulations, particularly the development of crystal-based long-acting injectable antipsychotics (LAIs).

New drugs – not a case of "me-tooism"

The development of truly novel antipsychotic treatments appears to have reached a plateau, marked by the disbanding of central nervous system research groups in some major pharmaceutical companies and the exhumation of previously discovered but undeveloped medications to fill the need for a broader palette of options. In this respect there may be some concern that the most recent developments are examples of "me-too" drugs, rather than those that add clinically meaningful depth to the pharmacopoeia. Essentially, the newer agents are serotonin/dopamine antagonists (SDAs) and thereby share a mode of action common to nearly all SGAs (exceptions include amisulpride). Furthermore, many of the "new" antipsychotics that are discussed in this chapter (eg, iloperidone, asenapine, lurasidone, and paliperidone) have been around for some time. Iloperidone, first developed in the early 1990s, has had an especially chequered pathway to US approval. Similarly, asenapine was developed in the early 1990s; and paliperidone is a primary metabolite of the long-standing antipsychotic staple risperidone, which has been available since 1993.

Despite this, it would be unwise to dismiss "me-too" drugs out of hand. There is little doubt that responsiveness can be a particularly individual matter in schizophrenia. Although, 30% of patients are likely to be refractory to standard treatments [72], there always exists the possibility that in any one particular person, there may be a match between the multireceptor targeting profile of newer drugs and the patient's particular neuropharmacological sensitivity, which may allow clozapine to be avoided. Although these agents are based on the centrality of dopamine antagonism as an essential component of their action – at least with respect to positive symptoms – their broader range of receptor affinities has been used to differentiate them in terms of tolerability and putative effectiveness with respect to other dimensional targets such as negative, cognitive, and affective symptoms. Apart from clozapine, any differences in positive symptom efficacy between the newer (atypical or SGA) medications and the FGAs is likely to be of marginal clinical significance. Effects at other targets may appear to be somewhat more robust, although apparent differences may be exaggerated by a combination of primary improvements through the manipulation of specific receptor interactions combined with the absence of more deleterious actions by the FGAs as they are discontinued. For example, the neuroleptic deficit syndrome along with akinesia and other immediate motor/cognitive effects might be considered a typical profile of FGAs. As these effects "wash out" and the newer, less toxic agents are added, emergent qualities of superior efficacy against cognitive deficits may actually reflect a different effect.

Although alternatives to direct dopamine and serotonin antagonism have been sought, such as agents acting on the glutamate pathways (see page 55), neuropeptide Y, serotonin receptor 2A antagonists, and many others, none have emerged as a replacement for the existing classes of SGAs. Some, as will be discussed, may have a role in adjunctive therapy, to target dimensions such as cognition and negative symptoms.

The following sections will first discuss the new oral antipsychotics, then some of the newer agents in early phase trials, and finally consider the role of LAIs, particularly the crystal-based agents (paliperidone palmitate and olanzapine pamoate).

Whether or not breakthrough drugs do emerge in the decades to come, their potential may still be undermined by one of the critical failures in psychiatric health care – that of ensuring adherence to treatment over the longer term.

Adverse events associated with specific receptor signaling

What can we expect from the new antipsychosis medications? Many antipsychotics come to market with a thorough Phase III testing period behind them. However, in many of these studies, which have been designed for the purposes of regulatory approval, there are particular limits on the populations studied. When the medication is released into the real clinical setting, physicians often determine what the "real world" average doses are, and what the main side effects experienced by the patients are likely to be for their typical cohort. Before clinicians are able to obtain such experience, it is often helpful to look at the preclinical pharmacology as this may help in identifying effects that may occur as a consequence of the interaction with various receptors. Figure 2.14

Clinical aspects of iloperidone, asenapine, and lurasidone

	ILO	ASEN	LUR
Indication*	Acute schizophrenia	Acute schizophrenia, maintenance schizophrenia, bipolar disorder	Acute schizophrenia
Dosing	BID	BID	OD
Formulations	Oral	Sublingual (do not swallow; no food for following 10 mins)	Oral (with food)
Up titration	4 days titration	Up to 7 days titration (maintenance)	To target dose
Metabolism	CYP2D6; 3A4	UGT1A4; CYP1A2A	CYP3A4
EPS	Flat/low	Dose dependent	Dose dependent
Sedation	Some	Most	Some (dose dependent)
Cardiac	Potential QTc effects	Low	Low
Weight/metabolics	Low/moderate	Low/moderate	Low

Figure 2.14 Clinical aspects of iloperidone, asenapine, and lurasidone. *Indication may differ by country/region. ASEN, asenapine; BD, twice daily; EPS, extrapyramidal symptoms; ILO, iloperidone; LUR, lurasidone; OD, once daily.

compares pharmacology of three recently released medications: asenapine, iloperidone, and lurasidone [73,74].

Figures 2.15 and 2.16 compare receptor affinities of various anti-psychotic medications and the clinical therapeutic and adverse effects that have been associated with various receptor types and are discussed in this section.

Weight gain

Kroeze et al provide evidence that the drugs most associated with weight gain are those that are antagonists of the histamine H_1 receptor and to a lesser extent α_1 adrenergic receptors [75]. There is also an association between the serotonin $5\text{-}HT_6$ and $5\text{-}HT_{2C}$ receptor antagonists or inverse agonists, although the latter by itself is not predictive of weight gain. Based on this model one could expect weight gain to occur in asenapine, paliperidone, and iloperidone to a greater extent than lurasidone. In the absence of long-standing use, the comparative rates of sequelae of weight gain such as the metabolic syndrome and diabetes, are not sufficiently established.

Extrapyramidal side effects

All new agents are SDAs and thus may be expected to have lower extrapyramidal symptoms (EPS) than FGAs. With no intrinsic anticholinergic effects (which may lessen apparent EPS) some "atypicality" may be afforded by a higher $5\text{-}HT_{2A}$ to D_2 receptor occupancy ratio (iloperidone)

Receptor affinities of various antipsychotic medications

	D_2	$5\text{-}HT_{2A}$	$5\text{-}HT_{2C}$	$5\text{-}HT_{1A}$	H_1	α_1	α_2	M_1	$5\text{-}HT_7$
Asenapine	+++	+++	++++	+++*	++	+++	+++	0	+++
Iloperidone	+++	++++	++	+	++	++++	+++	0	
Lurasidone	+++	+++	±	+++*	0	±	+	0	++++
Paliperidone	+++	+++	±	±	++	++	±	0	
Sertindole	+++	++++	+++	±	±	+++	±	0	
Clozapine	±	+++	+++	+*	+++	+++	+++	+++	±
Olanzapine	++	+++	++	0	++++	++	±	++	
Risperidone	+++	++++	+	±	+++	+++	++	0	+++
Haloperidol	+++	±	0	0	±	++	±	0	0

Figure 2.15 Receptor affinities of various antipsychotic medications. *Partial agonism. 5-HT, serotonin; α, adrenergic; D, dopamine; H, histamine; M, muscarinic.

Therapeutic and adverse effects of binding to target receptor

Receptor	Therapeutic	Adverse
D_2, D_3	• Reduces positive symptoms	• EPS: dystonia, parkinsonism, akathisia, tardive dystonia, rabbit syndrome • Neurohormonal (hyperprolactinemia) • NIDS
D_1	• Increases PFC function (agonism)	• Cognitive effects (antagonism)
α_1	• Improves cognition under high stress	• Postural hypotension, dizziness, reflex tachycardia • Potentiates hypotensive effect of prazosin • May enhance weight gain
α_2	• May potentiate antipsychotic effects and reduce EPS	• Blocks antihypertensive effect of clonidine
H_1	• Sedation (acute, short-term use only)	• Sedation, drowsiness, weight gain
M_1 (antagonism)	• Reduces EPS	• Memory effects (dysmnesia)
M_1 (agonism)	• Improves cognition	• Not known
$5\text{-HT}_{2A/2C}$	• Reduces EPS • Improves cognition and reduces negative symptoms	• Weight gain (5-HT_{2C} in association with other receptors)
5-HT_{7}	• Ameliorates depression; improves cognition	• Not known
5-HT_{1A} (agonism)	• Enhanced dopamine release in PFC and motor areas • Anti-aggressive, anxiolytic, and mood stabilizing	• Worsens EPS in full agonism
NMDA complex	• Cognitive (agonist)	• Neurotoxicity, psychosis

Figure 2.16 Therapeutic and adverse effects of binding to target receptor. 5-HT, serotonin; α, adrenergic; D, dopamine; EPS, extrapyramidal symptoms; NIDS, neuroleptic deficit syndrome; NMDA, N-methyl-D-aspartate; PFC, prefrontal cortex.

and the possible influence of potent α_2 antagonism (eg, asenapine, iloperidone). There may also be an effect from partial 5-HT_{1A} agonism (eg, asenapine, lurasidone), which putatively may reduce EPS through a reduction in raphe to striatum serotonergic tone.

Sedation

Whereas physicians tend to rate weight gain and EPS as being more important than sedation, it is the latter that patients and their families often complain about. Aside from management of an acute relapse, complaints of sedation should be taken seriously and attempts made to lessen this side effect. Based on the pharmacology of asenapine and iloperidone, these drugs could be expected to be more sedative than lurasidone due to H_1 and α_1 blockade. Early reports, however, suggest that asenapine has the most sedation, followed by iloperidone and (dose dependently) lurasidone. Like all side effects that are influenced by multiple endogenous and exogenous conditions, this will require individual assessment in the clinic. Other side effects of note for each medicine can be found in early reviews.

Similarly, comparative efficacy can be estimated to some degree from these reports. Lurasidone has been studied using olanzapine as an active comparator. Essentially there was no difference in efficacy between lurasidone (40–120 mg/day) and olanzapine 15 mg/day, although there were differences in the range and degree of side effects, particularly weight gain, favoring lurasidone [76,77]. Asenapine trials have mainly been short-term and placebo-controlled studies. When olanzapine was used as an active comparator (not a direct head-to-head comparator), asenapine showed a similar to somewhat lower efficacy profile depending on how the results are interpreted. Iloperidone has been trialed by active comparators, but no studies were clearly designed as head-to-head comparisons (rather, placebo was the main comparator). Similarly, these findings do not answer the question of whether the symptom efficacy is on par with standard medications, although there is no doubt that they perform better than placebo. At this early stage of clinical use, postmarketing studies should be expected, where head-to-head comparisons are performed with well-established agents in appropriately selected populations and are sufficiently well-powered.

At the same time it is important not to focus on the nominal class of agent (FGAs vs SGAs), as this distinction has become somewhat vague. In keeping with the dictum that all treatment should be individualized, this approach should push clinicians toward examining the risks and benefits of each medication and tailoring them to the individual's specific need and/or vulnerability to adverse effects.

Agents targeting the metabotropic glutamate system

Brief mention should be made of the metabotropic glutamate receptor (mGluR) agonists and positive allosteric modulators. Group I mGluRs (mGluR1 and 5) are located postsynaptically, where they may play a role in modulating both glutamate and dopamine neurotransmission. Group II mGluRs (mGluR2 and 3) are found presynaptically, and are thought to directly modulate the release of glutamate. These agents could be considered to be a new generation of treatment due to their very different pharmacological targets when compared to dopamine antagonists and inverse agonists (ie, standard antipsychotics). A full description of progress in the development of these agents is beyond the scope of this chapter, however, a brief summary of research to date will be presented.

Whereas the precise mechanisms by which mGluR agonists and positive allosteric modulators may be effective in schizophrenia has not been elucidated, an early proof of concept trial of an mGlu2/3 agonist showed promise. A more recent and larger study in patients with schizophrenia was deemed "inconclusive" as neither the study agent nor the active comparator (olanzapine) could be differentiated from placebo. Clearly, further studies using mGluR agonists are required.

It can be argued that positive allosteric modulators may be closer to the "physiological state," in that they may increase the effect of the natural ligand but only when it is binding to the orthostatic site. Although such agents are under development, none have received extensive investigation in patients with schizophrenia to date. It is useful to keep these agents in mind, as they may provide a method of targeting specific deficits (eg, cognition, motivation) when used as part of rational polypharmacy with antidopaminergics. However, early toxic outcomes (eg, seizures) in patients receiving mGluR2/3 agonists suggest that very careful attention should be paid to the risk–benefit ratio of these agents.

Form versus formulation

As discussed in the chapter on adherence, the actual effectiveness of medication may be a function of the patient's understanding of the costs and benefits of their treatment, a realization of whether they have an illness, and how intense it is, as well as the known efficacy and tolerability of the medicine. All of these factors influence the patient's preference and thus the rate of adherence (Figure 2.17). No matter how good or poor a medication is on paper, it will not help if the patient does not take it.

Although the new SDA-based medicines do not appreciably change the paradigm of antipsychotic action, immediate outcome gains can be made by improving the adherence to treatment, thereby enhancing the overall clinical effectiveness. For this reason antipsychotic formulation has become a mainstream clinical issue. As shown in Figure 2.18, for most oral medications, nonadherence is covert and it is difficult to detect without objective tests such as therapeutic drug monitoring. The next best strategy involves using the medication possession ratio, although this might not be suitable in all service delivery contexts.

To make nonadherence overt, the use of LAIs is the most effective way of knowing when a patient is receiving their medication (or not, depending on the service structure). In the case of direct medication supervision, dissolvable tablets offer the next best avenue of ensuring that the medicine is likely to have been ingested. A similar case can be made for liquid forms, such as for risperidone. If tablets or capsules have to be used, than persistent adherence is much more likely if there is a simple medication regimen (eg, once daily, at a time that allows for any peak side effects to occur during sleep). Additionally, the once-daily medication may be beneficial if it can be taken independently of food, a potential problem when prescribing ziprasidone and lurasidone, for example. As side effects may contribute to a patient's negative assessment of a medication, providing mechanisms to reduce the difference between high peak to trough levels seen with most oral medications may be useful. The OROS® technology used with paliperidone capsules flattens the daily peak–trough profile and may contribute to the low overall rate of EPS.

Of the new medications discussed here, paliperidone has both the OROS once-daily technology for oral delivery, and a newer crystal-based LAI form. Asenapine is administered by a sublingual tablet. However, asenapine and iloperidone are given twice daily, whereas lurasidone is given once daily, but must be taken with food. In other words, the kinetic profile affects delivery of the medication, which in turn may impair

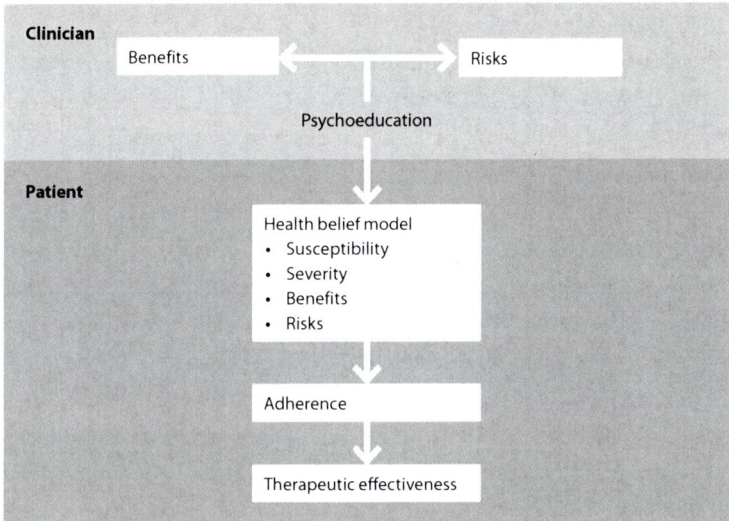

Figure 2.17 The views of clinicians and patients on therapeutic effectiveness of treatment.

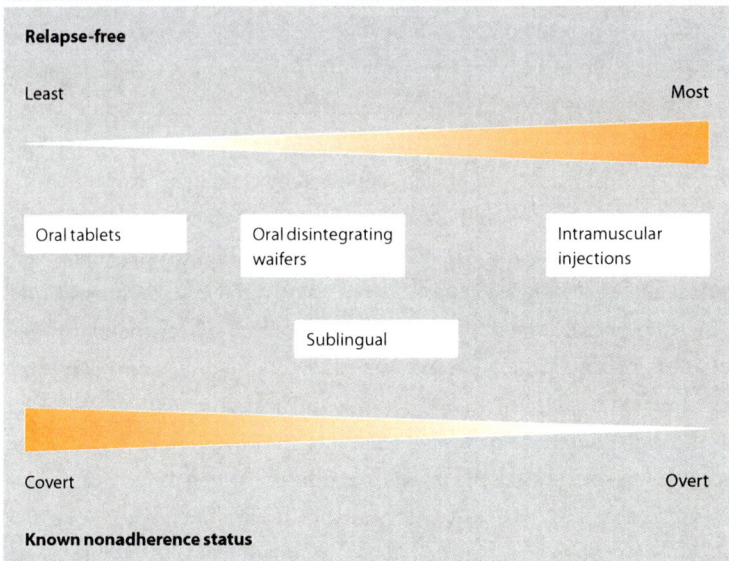

Figure 2.18 Relationship between nonadherence and relapse.

effectiveness through poor adherence if there is no adequate external medication-taking support.

New developments in the use of long-acting antipsychotics in the treatment of schizophrenia

As discussed elsewhere in this chapter (see page 27), rates of non- and partial adherence in schizophrenia are very high, with about two-thirds of patients missing significant amounts of oral medication in any 12-month period [78]. LAI antipsychotics have been developed with the aim of improving the long-term treatment of schizophrenia, primarily through improving the parlous rates of nonadherence. Relative to older antipsychotics, more recently developed antipsychotics combine variable efficacy at a broader range of targets with improved motor, neuro-cognitive, and neurohormonal tolerability. Long-acting forms of these agents might therefore be expected to combine better adherence with the benefits associated with the new generation agents. Whilst it should be emphasized that antipsychotic medication forms the key part of an individualized comprehensive treatment plan, which should include psychosocial interventions, a detailed discussion of the nonpharmacological management of schizophrenia is beyond the scope of this section, which reviews the use of LAIs in the practical management of schizophrenia.

Various lines of evidence support the use of LAIs, also known as "depots." These include randomized controlled trials, open studies, and mirror studies, which are further supported by comparing continuous to intermittent therapy as well as by expert opinion in most clinical practice guidelines. In the recent ADHERE study, LAIs demonstrated improved patient adherence when compared to oral antipsychotics (97.7% vs 42.3%) [79]. Differentially high LAI adherence rates have also been found in other settings, including the USA and Australia. The regular administration schedule of LAIs also facilitates rapid identification of patients who are overtly nonadherent, allowing clinicians to determine whether suboptimal treatment responses are due to a lack of efficacy or nonadherence issues.

There are now three SGA LAIs available in the clinic: risperidone LAI (RLAI), olanzapine pamoate LAI (OLAI), and paliperidone palmitate LAI

(PLAI). An overview of these agents can be found in Figure 2.19, which shows that there is a number of differences between the formulations, including the need for initiation/loading strategies, requirements for oral supplementation to offset the time to steady state, time to onset of antipsychotic actions, range of injection frequencies, sites of injection, mechanical issues of storage and reconstitution, and the need for special precautions.

Comparison of second-generation antipsychotic long-acting injections

	RLAI	PLAI	OLAI
Formulation	• Microsphere	• Crystal	• Crystal
Initiation/loading strategy	• Not possible	• Yes: day 1, then day 8, then monthly	• Yes: variable, depends on oral equivalence target
Requires oral supplementation	• Yes: 3+ weeks if switching from oral; • No: if switching from LAI	• No	• Not usually
Onset of clinical effect	• ≥4–5 weeks	• ≤1 week	• ≤1 week
Injection frequency	• 2-weekly	• Once-monthly	• 2- or 4-weekly§
Injection site	• Gluteal; deltoid*	• Deltoid; gluteal	• Gluteal
Reconstitution	• Powder in vial	• Prefilled syringes	• Powder in vial
Storage	• Refrigerated	• Room temp	• Room temp
Available doses*	• 25, 37.5, 50 mg	• 25, 50, 75, 100, 150 mg†	• 210, 300, 405 mg
Special precautions	• Take out of the fridge 30 minutes before use	• None	• Postinjection syndrome; requires mandatory 3-hour observation and transport protocols to be in place*,‡

Figure 2.19 Comparison of second-generation antipsychotic long-acting injections.
*Availability may differ by country; †in the USA PLAI doses are shown as paliperidone palmitate and so the equivalences to those in the table are 39, 78, 117, 156, 234 mg, respectively; ‡protocols may reflect what an allowable facility entails, who will monitor, who will take the patient to and from the injection facility, and procedures for dealing with the postinjection syndrome, if it occurs; §to achieve an equivalence of 20 mg/day of oral olanzapine, no 4-weekly OLAI dose is approved at present. OLAI, olanzapine long-acting injection; PLAI, paliperidone long-acting injection; RLAI, risperidone long-acting injection. Adapted from Haddad et al [80].

Paliperidone palmitate

Paliperidone is the major active metabolite of risperidone and the palmitate ester of paliperidone and is one of only two crystal-based LAIs available at present. PLAI crystals are provided in an aqueous, rather than an oil-based, suspension that utilizes nanoparticle technology. There are many advantages to using crystal-based LAIs: primarily their onset of action is usually within the first week (as with oral antipsychotics). Thus, treatment may be commenced in situations of acute relapses, and the effectiveness of the treatment may be established even after short administration periods, which is in distinct contrast to FGA LAIs and RLAI that have a lag period before providing sufficient antipsychotic release without oral supplementation. Furthermore, this agent can be administered in either the deltoid or the gluteal muscles, and in fact allows for some control of the release kinetics depending on the injection site (deltoid has a greater C_{max} and is recommended for at least the first two loading doses). The structure of the nanoparticles allows for a relatively long apparent half-life and the standard injection frequency is monthly.

Although efficacy data on PLAI are limited at this time, an intramuscular gluteal injection of long-acting paliperidone was shown to be significantly more effective than placebo in treating a first episode of schizophrenia in two double-blind, randomized studies. In 518 patients with schizophrenia, once monthly PLAI administered over 13 weeks produced clinically meaningful improvements across all efficacy measures: positive and negative syndrome scale total ($P<0.001$ vs placebo), positive and negative symptom scores ($P\leq0.05$), and clinical global impression severity scores ($P\leq0.006$) [81]. These findings have been confirmed in a 9-week study in which the PLAI responder rate (without oral supplementation) was 2.5-fold higher than that of placebo (37% vs 14% with $\geq30\%$ improvement in positive and negative syndrome scale total score) [82]. Relative to placebo, PLAI was generally well tolerated with a similar incidence of treatment-emergent events and low rates of EPS (5% vs 6%) [82]. In another placebo-controlled recurrence prevention study, PLAI significantly delayed time to relapse compared with placebo, without unexpected adverse events [82]. Although head-to-head comparative trials will be needed to confirm these results, the efficacy and tolerability of paliperidone support its use as a viable treatment option in the acute management of psychosis. This is a game-changing development considering that older depots did not allow for an effective and safe acute use strategy.

To date, few studies have investigated the efficacy of SGA LAIs in the prevention of relapse as a primary clinical end point. However, available data indicate that SGA LAIs significantly reduce relapse rates. PLAI appears to be effective in relapse prevention. In a 6-month "real-world" study in stabilized patients with schizophrenia (n=408), PLAI significantly delayed the time to relapse (P<0.0001) and produced a threefold reduction in the rate of relapse (10% vs 34% for placebo) [83]. Studies of longer duration are expected for PLAI in order to establish its long-term effectiveness.

PLAI may also play an important role in helping to differentiate those with resistance to treatment versus true treatment-refractory schizophrenia. The former implies the possibility of modifiable reasons for poor outcome, whereas the latter suggests that adequate treatment has been applied (ie, medications have reached their target receptors in optimal concentrations for optimal periods, and appropriate psychosocial interventions transacted), but there has been little or insufficient response. After examining various resistance-to-treatment factors, it is common to find that adherence to past treatments cannot be confirmed. This leads to an important question as to whether the so-called resistance to treatment was simply inadequate effectiveness due to nonadherence.

Ultimately, the only sure test of whether adherence issues are at the root of the poor outcomes is to ensure adherence through a trial of an LAI. A priori end-points should be defined in order to gauge the success of LAI intervention. Preceding such a trial, the following factors should be established: (i) the trial time frame; (ii) symptoms or outcome dimensions that are expected to improve; (iii) how the symptoms should be measured and by whom; and (iv) the minimal/threshold shifts required to determine drug responsiveness. By setting the threshold for improvement in a manner that is readily discernible by the treatment team, it usually becomes clear within 3 months whether LAI is having an effect, although up to 5 or 6 months may be required in some cases. For those who respond, continuing maintenance with LAI is recommended, while issues of adherence to oral treatments are addressed. However, when patients show no response and treatment-refractory disease seems likely, it is important to switch to clozapine as soon as possible. Delays in the initiation of clozapine may lead to less robust responses, and maintaining LAI treatment with no real therapeutic benefit and many potential risks poses ethical concerns.

Advantages of PLAI in the clinic

Not all benefits of new medications and formulations lie in the pharmacology alone. In case of PLAI, the following may facilitate its use in overstretched community psychiatric settings and thereby enhance the efficiency of services:

- injections once every month;
- no special storage requirements such as cold chain;
- different needle sizes available for varying patient body-mass index;
- provision of prefilled syringes with no need to spend time preparing a suspension;
- deltoid or gluteal injections (although not researched adequately to date, the ability to give the injection in the deltoid may also be seen as an advantage for quicker, less stigmatizing delivery, both from the patient's and service's points of view);
- no 3-hour observation period required;
- no requirement to monitor transport to and from the injecting facility;
- may be given anywhere (eg, patient's home, work, office).

Conclusion

This section has reviewed medications for schizophrenia that have been recently released as well as those approaching release. Whereas the newer oral antidopaminergic agents do not have new mechanisms of action (being SDA drugs), their broader range of effects at key receptors allows their overall cost–benefit profile to be sufficiently different. The individualization of treatment requires a broad palette of options when treating schizophrenia, and new agents may "work" in particular cases where others have failed. Such targeted multireceptor approaches may be effective through a "magic shotgun" approach, rather than that of a "magic bullet."

The problem of nonadherence underlies all management of chronic disease states. The acceptance of, and the direct approach to, managing such states increasingly lies with new formulations of existing medications that clearly highlight overt nonadherence. Crystal-based LAIs may represent one of the advantages of new delivery systems providing better adherence and outcomes in the longer term.

References

1 McGlashan T, Walsh B, Woods S. *The Psychosis-Risk Syndrome Handbook for Diagnosis and Follow-Up*. New York, NY: Oxford University Press; 2010.

2 Schultze-Lutter F, Michel C, Ruhrmann S, Klosterkötter J, Schimmelmann BG. Prediction and early detection of first-episode psychosis. In: Ritsner M, ed. *Textbook of Schizophrenia Spectrum Disorders, Volume II*. Dordrecht, the Netherlands: Springer Science + Business Media; 2011:207-268.

3 The American Psychiatric Association DSM-5 development: proposed draft revisions to DSM disorders and criteria. www.dsm5.org/ProposedRevision/Pages/Default.aspx. Accessed April 2, 2012.

4 Carpenter WT Jr. Criticism of the DSM-V risk syndrome: a rebuttal. *Cogn Neuropsychiatry*. 2011;16:101-106.

5 Miller TJ, McGlashan TH, Rosen JL, et al. Prospective diagnosis of the initial prodrome for schizophrenia based on the structured interview for prodromal syndromes: preliminary evidence of interrater reliability and predictive validity. *Am J Psychiatry*. 2002;159:863-865.

6 Yung AR, Phillips LJ, Yuen HP, et al. Psychosis prediction: 12-month follow up of a high-risk ("prodromal") group. *Schizophr Res*. 2003;60:21-32.

7 Yung AR, Phillips LJ, Yuen HP, McGorry PD. Risk factors for psychosis in an ultra high-risk group: psychopathology and clinical features. *Schizophr Res*. 2004; 67:131-142.

8 Haroun N, Dunn L, Haroun A, Cadenhead KS. Risk and protection in prodromal schizophrenia: ethical implications for clinical practice and future research. *Schizophr Bull*. 2006;32:166-178.

9 Cannon TD, Cadenhead K, Cornblatt B, et al. Prediction of psychosis in youth at high clinical risk: a multisite longitudinal study in North America. *Arch Gen Psychiatry*. 2008;65:28-37.

10 Ruhrmann S, Schultze-Lutter F, Salokangas RK, et al. Prediction of psychosis in adolescents and young adults at high risk: results from the prospective European prediction of psychosis study. *Arch Gen Psychiatry*. 2010;67:241-251.

11 Simon AE, Umbricht D. High remission rates from an initial ultra-high risk state for psychosis. *Schizophr Res*. 2010;116:168-172.

12 Addington J, Cornblatt BA, Cadenhead KS, et al. At clinical high risk for psychosis: outcome for nonconverters. *Am J Psychiatry*. 2011;168:800-805.

13 Yung AR, Yuen HP, McGorry PD, et al. Mapping the onset of psychosis: the Comprehensive Assessment of At-Risk Mental States. *Aust N Z J Psychiatry*. 2005;39:964-971.

14 Schultze-Lutter F, Klosterkötter J Picker H, Steinmeyer EM, Ruhrmann S. Predicting first-episode psychosis by basic symptom criteria. *Clin Neuropsych*. 2007;4:11-22.

15 Schultze-Lutter F, Ruhrmann S, Klosterkötter J. Can schizophrenia be predicted phenomenologically? In: Johannesen JO, Martindale BV, Cullberg J, eds. *Evolving Psychosis: Different Stages, Different Treatments*. Hove, UK: Routledge; 2006:104-123.

16 Klosterkötter J, Hellmich M, Steinmeyer EM, Schultze-Lutter F. Diagnosing schizophrenia in the initial prodromal phase. *Arch Gen Psychiatry*. 2001;58:158-164.

17 Klosterkötter J, Ruhrmann S, Schultze-Lutter F, et al. The European Prediction of Psychosis Study (EPOS): integrating early recognition and intervention in Europe. *World Psychiatry*. 2005;4:161-167.

18 Klosterkötter J, Schultze-Lutter F, Bechdolf A, Ruhrmann S. Prediction and prevention of schizophrenia: what has been achieved and where to go next? *World Psychiatry*. 2011;10:165-174.

19 Fusar-Poli P, Bonoldi I, Yung AR, et al. Predicting psychosis: a meta-analysis of evidence. *Arch Gen Psychiatry*. In press.

20 Koch E, Schultze-Lutter F, Schimmelmann BG, Resch F. On the importance and detection of prodromal symptoms from the perspective of child and adolescent psychiatry. *Clin Neuropsych*. 2010;7:38-48.

21 American Psychiatric Association. Diagnostic and Statistical Manual of Mental Disorders (Text Revision). 4th edn. Washington, DC: American Psychiatric Press; 1994.

22 Preti A, Cella M. Randomized-controlled trials in people at ultra high risk of psychosis: a review of treatment effectiveness. *Schizophr Res*. 2010;123:30-36.

23 McGlashan TH, Zipursky RB, Perkins D, et al. Randomized, double-blind trial of olanzapine versus placebo in patients prodromally symptomatic for psychosis. *Am J Psychiat*. 2006;163:790-799.

24 McGorry PD, Yung AR, Phillips LJ, et al. Randomized controlled trial of interventions designed to reduce the risk of progression to first-episode psychosis in a clinical sample with subthreshold symptoms. *Arch Gen Psychiat*. 2002;59:921-928.

25 Morrison AP, French P, Walford L, et al. Cognitive therapy for the prevention of psychosis in people at ultra-high risk: randomised controlled trial. *Brit J Psychiat*. 2004;185:291-297.

26 Bechdolf A, Wagner M, Ruhrmann S, et al. Preventing progression to first-episode psychosis in early initial prodromal states. *Br J Psychiatry*. 2012;200:22-29.

27 Ruhrmann S, Bechdolf A, Kühn KU, et al. Acute effects of treatment for prodromal symptoms for people putatively in a late initial prodromal state of psychosis. *Br J Psychiatry*. 2007;191(suppl 51):s88-s95.

28 Amminger GP, Schäfer MR, Klier CM, et al. Decreased nervonic acid levels in erythrocyte membranes predict psychosis in help-seeking ultra-high-risk individuals. *Mol Psychiatry*. 2011. [Epub ahead of print].

29 International Early Psychosis Association Writing Group. International clinical practice guidelines for early psychosis. *Br J Psychiatry Suppl*. 2005;48:s120-s124.

30 McGorry P, Killackey E, Elkins K, Lambert M, Lambert T. Summary Australian and New Zealand clinical practice guideline for the treatment of schizophrenia (2003). *Australasian Psych*. 2003;11:136-147.

31 Ventura J, Hellemann GS, Thames AD, Koellner V, Nuechterlein KH. Symptoms as mediators of the relationship between neurocognition and functional outcome in schizophrenia: a meta-analysis. *Schizophr Res*. 2009;113:189-199.

32 Moritz S, Woodward TS. Metacognitive training in schizophrenia: from basic research to knowledge translation and intervention. *Curr Opin Psychiatry*. 2007;20:619-625.

33 Caldwell C, Gottesman I. Schizophrenics kill themselves too: a review of risk factors for suicide. *Schizophr Bull*. 1990;16:571-589.

34 Limosin F, Loze JY, Philippe A, Casadebaig F, Rouillon F. Ten-year prospective follow-up study of the mortality by suicide in schizophrenic patients. *Schizophrenia Research*. 2007;94:23-28.

35 Stephens J, Richard P, McHugh PR. Suicide in patients hospitalized for schizophrenia: 1913-1940. *J Nerv Ment Dis*. 1999;187:10-14.

36 Tanney BL. Psychiatric diagnoses and suicidal acts. In: Maris RW, Berman AL, Silverman MM, eds. *Comprehensive Textbook of Suicidology*. New York, NY: Guilford Press; 2000: 311-341.

37 Harkavy-Friedman JM, Nelson EA. Assessment and intervention for the suicidal patient with schizophrenia. *Psychiatr Q*. 1997;68:361-375.

38 Kallert TW, Leisse M, Winiecki P. Suicidality of chronic schizophrenic patients in long-term community care. *Crisis*. 2004;25:54-64.

39 Fenton WS. Depression, suicide, and suicide prevention in schizophrenia. *Suicide Life Threat Behav*. 2000;30:34-49.

40 Robinson J, Cotton S, Conus P, Schimmelmann BG, McGorry P, Lambert M. Prevalence and predictors of suicide attempt in an incidence cohort of 661 young people with first-episode psychosis. *Aust N Z J Psychiatry*. 2009;43:149-157.

41 Power PJ, Bell RJ, Mills R, et al. Suicide prevention in first episode psychosis: the development of a randomised controlled trial of cognitive therapy for acutely suicidal patients with early psychosis. *Aust N Z J Psychiatry*. 2003;37:414-420.

42 Velligan DI, Weiden PJ, Sajatovic M, et al. The expert consensus guideline series: adherence problems in patients with serious and persistent mental illness. *J Clin Psychiatry*. 2009;70(suppl 4):1-46.

43 Lambert M, Conus P, Cotton S, Robinson J, McGorry PD, Schimmelmann BG. Prevalence, predictors, and consequences of long-term refusal of antipsychotic treatment in first-episode psychosis. *J Clin Psychopharmacol*. 2010;30:565-572.

44 Conus P, Lambert M, Cotton S, Bonsack C, McGorry PD, Schimmelmann BG. Rate and predictors of service disengagement in an epidemiological first-episode psychosis cohort. *Schizophr Res*. 2010;118:256-263.

45 Schimmelmann BG, Conus P, Schacht M, McGorry P, Lambert M. Predictors of service disengagement in first-admitted adolescents with psychosis. *J Am Acad Child Adolesc Psychiatry*. 2006;45:990-999.

46 Velligan DI, Lam YW, Glahn DC, et al. Defining and assessing adherence to oral antipsychotics: a review of the literature. *Schizophr Bull*. 2006;32:724-742.

47 Lacro JP, Dunn LB, Dolder CR, Leckband SG, Jeste DV. Prevalence of and risk factors for medication nonadherence in patients with schizophrenia: a comprehensive review of recent literature. *J Clin Psychiatry*. 2002;63:892-909.

48 Goff DC, Hill M, Freudenreich O. Strategies for improving treatment adherence in schizophrenia and schizoaffective disorder. *J Clin Psychiatry*. 2010; 71(suppl 2):20-26.

49 President's Commission for the Study of Ethical Problems in Medicine and Biomedical and Behavioral Research. bioethics.georgetown.edu/pcbe/reports/past_commissions/making_health_care_decisions.pdf. Accessed April 2, 2012.

50 Makoul G, Clayman ML. An integrative model of shared decision making in medical encounters. *Patient Educ Couns*. 2006;60:301-312.

51 Xia J, Merinder LB, Belgamwar MR. Psychoeducation for schizophrenia. *Cochrane Database Syst Rev*. 2011;(6):CD002831.

52 de Leon J, Dadvand M, Canuso C, White AO, Stanilla JK, Simpson GM. Schizophrenia and smoking: an epidemiological survey in a state hospital. *Am J Psychiatry*. 1995;152:453-455.

53 Hughes JR, Hatsukami DK, Mitchell JE, Dahlgren LA. Prevalence of smoking among psychiatric outpatients. *Am J Psychiatry*. 1986;143:993-997.

54 Goff DC, Henderson DC, Amico E. Cigarette smoking in schizophrenia: relationship to psychopathology and medication side effects. *Am J Psychiatry*. 1992;149:1189-1194.

55 Yarnold PR, Levinson DF, Singh H, et al. Prevalence of substance abuse in schizophrenia: demographic and clinical correlates. *Schizophr Bull*. 1990;16:31-56.

56 Barnett JH, Werners U, Secher SM, et al. Substance use in a population-based clinic sample of people with first-episode psychosis. *Br J Psychiatry*. 2007;190:515-520.

57 Mauri MC, Volonteri LS, De Gaspari IF, Colasanti A, Brambilla MA, Cerruti L. Substance abuse in first-episode schizophrenic patients: a retrospective study. *Clin Pract Epidemiol Ment Health*. 2006;2:4.

58 Kuepper R, van Os J, Lieb R, Wittchen HU, Höfler M, Henquet C. Continued cannabis use and risk of incidence and persistence of psychotic symptoms: 10 year follow-up cohort study. *BMJ*. 2011;342:d738.

59 Meister K, Burlon M, Rietschel L, Gouzoulis-Mayfrank E, Bock T, Lambert M. [Dual diagnosis psychosis and substance use disorders in adolescents – part 1]. *Fortschr Neurol Psychiatr*. 2010;78:81-89.

60 Meister K, Rietschel L, Burlon M, Gouzoulis-Mayfrank E, Bock T, Lambert M. [Dual diagnosis psychosis and substance use disorders in adolescents – part 2]. *Fortschr Neurol Psychiatr.* 2010;78:90-100.

61 Morgan C, Fisher H. Environment and schizophrenia: environmental factors in schizophrenia: childhood trauma – a critical review. *Schizophr Bull.* 2007;33:3-10.

62 Janssen I, Krabbendam L, Bak M, et al. Childhood abuse as a risk factor for psychotic experiences. *Acta Psychiatr Scand.* 2004;109:38-45.

63 Kessler RC, Chiu WT, Demler O, Merikangas KR, Walters EE. Prevalence, severity, and comorbidity of 12-month DSM-IV disorders in the National Comorbidity Survey Replication. *Arch Gen Psychiatry.* 2005;62:617-627.

64 Gearon JS, Kaltman SI, Brown C, Bellack AS. Traumatic life events and PTSD among women with substance use disorders and schizophrenia. *Psychiatr Serv.* 2003;54:523-528.

65 Fan X, Henderson DC, Nguyen DD, et al. Posttraumatic stress disorder, cognitive function and quality of life in patients with schizophrenia. *Psychiatry Res.* 2008;159:140-146.

66 Quarantini LC, Miranda-Scippa A, Nery-Fernandes F, et al. The impact of comorbid posttraumatic stress disorder on bipolar disorder patients. *J Affect Disord.* 2010;123:71-76.

67 Goldberg JF, Garno JL. Development of posttraumatic stress disorder in adult bipolar patients with histories of severe childhood abuse. *J Psychiatr Res.* 2005;39:595-601.

68 Read J. Breaking the silence: learning why, when and how to ask about trauma, and how to respond to disclosure. In Larkin W, Morrisons A, eds. *Trauma and Psychosis.* London, UK: Brunner-Routledge; 2006:195-221.

69 Frueh BC, Grubaugh AL, Cusack KJ, Kimble MO, Elhai JD, Knapp RG. Exposure-based cognitive-behavioral treatment of PTSD in adults with schizophrenia or schizoaffective disorder: a pilot study. *J Anxiety Disord.* 2009;23:665-675.

70 Van den Berg DPG, van der Gaag M. Treating trauma in psychosis with EMDR: a pilot study. *J Behav Ther Exp Psychiatry.* 2012;43:664-671.

71 Mueser KT, Rosenberg SD, Xie H, et al. A randomized controlled trial of cognitive-behavioral treatment for posttraumatic stress disorder in severe mental illness. *J Consult Clin Psychol.* 2008;76:259-71.

72 Lambert TJ. Disease management: multidimensional approaches to incomplete recovery in psychosis. In Elkis H, Meltzer HY, eds. *Therapy-Resistant Schizophrenia.* Basel, Switzerland: Karger; 2010:87-113.

73 Citrome L. Iloperidone, asenapine, and lurasidone: a brief overview of 3 new second-generation antipsychotics. *Postgrad Med.* 2011;123:153-162.

74 McIntyre RS. Asenapine: a review of acute and extension phase data in bipolar disorder. *CNS Neurosci Ther.* 2011;17:645-648.

75 Kroeze WK, Hufeisen SJ, Popadak BA, et al. H1-histamine receptor affinity predicts short-term weight gain for typical and atypical antipsychotic drugs. *Neuropsychopharmacology.* 2003;28:519-526.

76 Loebel A, Cucchiaro J, Ogasa M, et al. Efficacy of lurasidone: summary of results from the clinical development program. Poster presented at: New Research Approaches to Mental Health Interventions (NCDEU) meeting; June 14-17, 2010; Boca Raton, FL.

77 Cucchiaro J, Silva R, Ogasa M, et al. Lurasidone in the treatment of acute schizophrenia: results of the double-blind, placebocontrolled PEARL 2 trial. *Schizophr Res.* 2010;117:493.

78 Williams CL, Johnstone BM, Kesterson JG, Javor KA, Schmetzer AD. Evaluation of antipsychotic and concomitant medication use patterns in patients with schizophrenia. *Med Care.* 1999;37(4 suppl Lilly):AS81-AS86.

79 Gutiérrez-Casares JR, Cañas F, Rodríguez-Morales A, Hidalgo-Borrajo R, Alonso-Escolano D. Adherence to treatment and therapeutic strategies in schizophrenic patients: the ADHERE study. *CNS Spectr.* 2010;15:327-337.

80 Haddad P, Lambert T, Lauriello J, eds. *Antipsychotic Long-Acting Injections.* New York, NY: Oxford University Press; 2011.

81 Nasrallah HA, Gopal S, Gassmann-Mayer C, et al. A controlled, evidence-based trial of paliperidone palmitate, a long-acting injectable antipsychotic, in schizophrenia. *Neuropsychopharmacology*. 2010;35:2072-2082.

82 Kramer M, Litman R, Hough D, et al. Paliperidone palmitate, a potential long-acting treatment for patients with schizophrenia. Results of a randomized, double-blind, placebo-controlled efficacy and safety study. *Int J Neuropsychopharmacol*. 2010;13:635-647.

83 Hough D, Gopal S, Vijapurkar U, Lim P, Morozova M, Eerdekens M. Paliperidone palmitate maintenance treatment in delaying the time-to-relapse in patients with schizophrenia: a randomized, double-blind, placebo-controlled study. *Schizophr Res*. 2010;116:107-117.

Organization of care and treatment

General principles of care

Martin Lambert and Dieter Naber

Good clinical practice

Good clinical practice requires a close, cooperative, and multidisciplinary treatment network for patients and relatives. The effects of schizophrenia on a patient's life can create such difficulties and impairments that multidisciplinary care providers have to work together closely. For professionals, three main requirements of good clinical practice across all phases of care are important:

1. shared knowledge of good clinical practice;
2. application of this knowledge into daily clinical practice; and
3. the same positive attitude toward possible success of treatment.

The guidelines of the National Institute for Health and Clinical Excellence (NICE), and other guidelines for schizophrenia (eg, the American, German, Canadian, and Australian guidelines for schizophrenia), have summarized recommendations for good clinical practice, attitude, and care in first- and multiple-episode psychosis [1–5]. The following principles should be considered:

- an optimistic attitude toward the patient with respect to outcome;
- providing effective treatment at the earliest possible opportunity;
- full assessment of the needs for health and social care;
- working in partnership with service users and carers;

M. Lambert and D. Naber, *Current Schizophrenia*,
DOI: 10.1007/978-1-908517-68-5_3,
© Springer Healthcare, a part of Springer Science+Business Media 2012

- supportive and understanding relationships between service users and carers;
- providing good information and mutual support;
- cooperation regarding the choice of treatment; and
- presence of a global treatment context.

Three major service components are linked to a better prognosis of schizophrenia:

1. Early detection and intervention in patients with prodromal psychosis with the goal of preventing or delay of the full manifestation of the disorder (also see Chapter 2).
2. Early detection and intervention in patients with first-episode psychosis (FEP) with the goal of reducing treatment delay and its negative consequences on outcome (also see Chapter 2).
3. High quality of care within all phases of illness.

Service requirements

Successful needs-adapted integrated care of patients with schizophrenia, regardless of whether in the prodromal, first-episode, or chronic phase, has specific service requirements, the most important of which are:

- Several institutions have to collaborate, including:
  - adult psychiatry and child and youth psychiatry for patients with prodrome or FEP with age-independent continuity of care or for patients with comorbid child and youth psychiatry disorders (eg, autism, Asperger's disorder);
  - geriatric psychiatry for older patients with psychosis and specifically for patients at risk for dementia;
  - a neuropsychology unit for neuropsychological testing;
  - a vocational therapy unit for specific vocational interventions such as supported employment;
  - patient and caregiver organizations, to discuss service structures and contents of treatment, implementation of experienced involvement, peer-to-peer and relatives-to-relatives support, and development of community educational materials and collaborative health education programs; and

- community mental health providers, such as private psychiatrists, psychologists, nurses, and housing facilities.
- Development of a catchment area for an early detection and treatment network, in which all collaborators work together and one early detection unit receives an assessment and treatment mandate from all network participants for the early detection and treatment of prodromal and first-episode patients.
- Within the psychosis center, implementation of inpatient, day clinic, and outpatient facilities. Services for prodromal and first-episode patients should be separated within an early detection and intervention center, including the implementation of an assertive early detection and intervention team. Attached to the outpatient center, an assertive community treatment center should be implemented. With respect to the outpatient center, teams for patients with schizophrenia-spectrum and bipolar disorder should be separated and should provide disease-specific interventions.
- Implementation of public health sector education, including stigma reduction strategies, targeted public education, and targeted service provider education. Such strategies have to be implemented long term as they lose the effects shortly after stopping them.
- Implementation of easy service access, including low referral threshold, single point of contact, acceptance of referrals from all sources, acceptance of patients with comorbid substance use disorder, and timely contact with referred individuals.
- Access to community support, including income support, housing support, community activities, and funding for medication.

A number of services that integrate these requirements have been developed. Representative specialized FEP programs can be found in Australia (ORYGEN Youth Health and Research Centre including the Early Psychosis Prevention and Intervention Centre) and Canada (Prevention and Early Intervention Program for Psychosis). Other services have included specialized prodromal and first-episode programs in a broader service structure (eg, Psychosis Early Detection and Intervention Center in the Psychosis Center at the University Medical Center, Hamburg, Germany; Figure 3.1).

Early detection and intervention in first-episode psychosis patients

Several potential benefits of early detection and early intervention in FEP have been discussed (see Chapter 2), and probably the most important ones are:

- reduction of the duration of the active psychotic phase; and
- reduction of delayed treatment in the active psychotic phase.

Both aspects are related to research on the so-called duration of untreated psychosis (DUP). Long DUP has been linked to several negative illness consequences:

- possibly a slower recovery or less complete recovery;
- a higher rate of hospitalization;
- an increased burden for relatives and other caregivers;
- an increased risk of damaging socioeconomic consequences;
- an increased risk of secondary comorbid problems, including substance abuse, suicide, and/or aggressive behavior;
- an increased risk of relapse;
- a reduction of functional level, including the possibility of worse functional outcome; and
- less positive short- and long-term prognosis.

The rationales and current guidelines of early detection and specialized treatment of patients with prodromal psychosis are described in Chapter 2.

Phase-specific treatments for schizophrenia

Martin Lambert and Dieter Naber

Treatments for schizophrenia are separated according to different phases of illness:

- the prodromal phase;
- the acute phase (including first- or recurrent multiple-episode); and
- the long-term phase (including a chronic illness or full or partial recovery).

Structure of the Psychosis Center at the Department of Psychiatry and Psychotherapy, University Medical Center, Hamburg, Germany

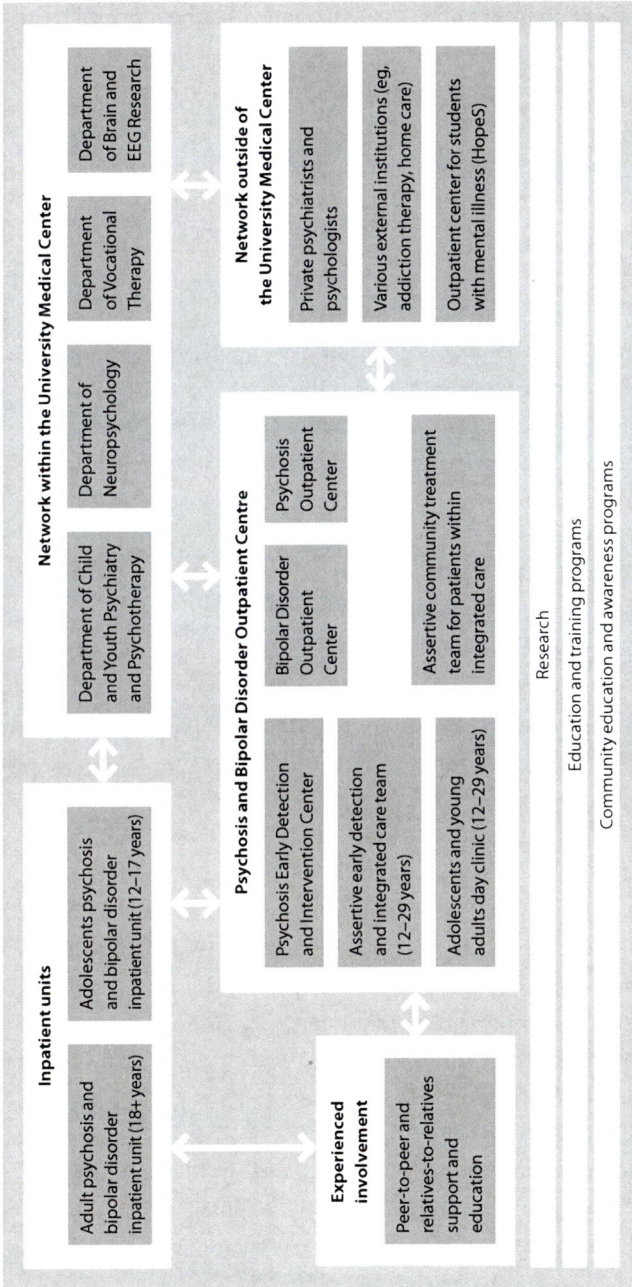

Inpatient units

Adult psychosis and bipolar disorder inpatient unit (18+ years)

Adolescents psychosis and bipolar disorder inpatient unit (12–17 years)

Network within the University Medical Center

Department of Child and Youth Psychiatry and Psychotherapy

Department of Neuropsychology

Department of Vocational Therapy

Department of Brain and EEG Research

Network outside of the University Medical Center

Private psychiatrists and psychologists

Various external institutions (eg, addiction therapy, home care)

Outpatient center for students with mental illness (HopeS)

Psychosis and Bipolar Disorder Outpatient Centre

Psychosis Early Detection and Intervention Center

Assertive early detection and integrated care team (12–29 years)

Adolescents and young adults day clinic (12–29 years)

Bipolar Disorder Outpatient Center

Psychosis Outpatient Center

Assertive community treatment team for patients within integrated care

Experienced involvement

Peer-to-peer and relatives-to-relatives support and education

Research

Education and training programs

Community education and awareness programs

Figure 3.1 Structure of the Psychosis Center at the Department of Psychiatry and Psychotherapy, University Medical Center, Hamburg, Germany. For more information see www.uke.de/kliniken/psychiatrie/index_40441.php

Across these phases of illness the following treatment principles should be applied:

- A strong working alliance with the patient and their relatives should be developed.
- The patient's initial discomfort should be minimized.
- Treatment should target a broad range of symptoms, comorbidities, and problems.
- Professional treatment should be continuous, and interruptions should be avoided.
- Interventions should be age- and stage-appropriate.
- The pace and timing of reintegration should be considered carefully.
- Family involvement should be regarded as being important.
- In the acute phase, behavioral emergencies should be separated from the usual acute treatment.

Treatment in the acute phase

Treatment in the acute phase has to be separated into acute treatment with and without behavioral emergency. This differentiation is needed because treatment guidelines for behavioral emergencies differ markedly from guidelines for "usual" acute treatment in schizophrenia. For treatment in the prodromal phase see Chapter 2 (page 13).

Goals of management of the acute phase

In the acute phase, the overall goals of management are (1) engagement and development of a therapeutic alliance with the patient and their family; (2) treatment of possible behavioral emergencies; (3) accomplishment of a comprehensive psychobiological assessment; (4) treatment of psychotic symptoms and possible comorbid symptoms/disorders; (5) formulation of an integrated short- and long-term treatment plan; and (6) connection of the patient with appropriate aftercare.

Engagement and development of a therapeutic alliance

Both the quality of the relationship with clinicians during the initial contact and the subsequent development of a trusting therapeutic alliance appear to be important determinants of a positive patient attitude toward treatment, adherence to medication, and overall treatment engagement. However, the initial engagement process can be damaged by a variety of factors, such as negative attitudes toward psychiatry, the current mental state of the patient (including behavioral disturbances, fears, suspiciousness, unawareness of the illness, cognitive problems in processing information, and concerns of the family and carers). Unfortunately, by the time of their first presentation, most patients have at least one of these complicating factors. Consequently, the first contact with the service is often critical, and engagement, initial assessment, and (early) treatment need to occur as a parallel process. Therefore, planning of the initial contact is important. All sources of information should be gathered before arranging the first assessment. This information will assist in choosing the most appropriate setting: the one with the highest chance of engagement, safety, and successful initiation of treatment. Well-trained and experienced staff, an individually adapted interview situation, and an appropriate interview technique are important requirements for successful first contact and assessment.

Treatment of behavioral disturbances

In the acute phase, an important treatment goal is to prevent and control acutely disturbed behaviors such as agitation, hostility, violence/aggression, pathological excitement, and suicidal ideation in a way that does not traumatize the patient and his or her family. A detailed overview is given later in this chapter (page 93).

Comprehensive psychobiological assessment

A comprehensive psychiatric investigation always comprises a number of psychosocial and neuromedical assessments. A neuropsychological assessment is recommended in prodromal and FEP patients as well as in patients with certain cognitive deficits that are clinically apparent. The identity of the psychotic disorder as well as possible comorbid psychiatric disorders should be determined on the basis of this information. A detailed overview is provided in Chapter 4 (page 166).

Treatment of psychotic symptoms and comorbid disorders

Treatment of psychotic symptoms and possible comorbid symptoms and disorders is the most important aspect of treatment in the acute phase. These interventions can be based at the hospital or carried out at home if safety is accurately addressed. A detailed overview is given later in this chapter.

Formulation of an integrated short- and long-term treatment plan

Another goal of acute treatment is the formulation of an individual phase- and stage-specific integrated treatment plan, which should be actively discussed with patients, relatives, and treatment providers in a shared decision-making process. The success of the previous plan of care, the present level of symptomatic remission, residual symptoms and functioning, social problems (eg, living situation), and risk factors affecting the success of the intended treatment plan (eg, risk of medication nonadherence or service disengagement) are the main factors on which an appropriate plan of care is based. Once the patient begins to recover, the goals of treatment – and thereby the therapeutic strategies – shift toward a more intense psychotherapeutic approach, with the goals of complete remission of symptoms, improvement in social functioning, and achievement of an adequate quality of life (see page 110). The vulnerability–stress–coping model provides a framework for integrating different therapeutic strategies and adapting interventions to the patient's functioning level.

Connecting the patient with appropriate aftercare

Connection with appropriate aftercare is an important challenge for patients with schizophrenia. It is complicated by the tendency of some patients to become directly disengaged from mental care services after inpatient treatment. Most appropriate is a link with an assertive community treatment team that has already become involved in the patient's care during inpatient treatment.

Principles of treatment to support successful pharmacotherapy in acute schizophrenia

- **Integrated care is required for optimal antipsychotic response.** Studies on incomplete remission and treatment resistance have shown that insufficient psychosocial intervention is a risk factor for poor response to antipsychotics and poor outcome.
- **Reduction of treatment delay improves response to antipsychotics.** Prolonged DUP, especially in combination with other response risk factors, seems to predict decreased response and poor outcome.
- **Treatment of comorbid psychiatric disorders may promote response.** Untreated and persistent comorbid psychiatric disorders are related to an increased risk of incomplete or no response. This was shown repeatedly for persistent substance abuse and is now also evident for comorbid disorders such as major depression, anxiety disorder, or personality disorder. In other words, untreated comorbidity lowers the chance of remission and recovery in schizophrenia. Second-generation antipsychotics (SGAs) are increasingly used as an add-on therapy for various nonpsychotic disorders, which is an argument for their first-line use.
- **Patients and relatives should participate in treatment planning.** The participation of patients in treatment planning is being increasingly advocated. The shared decision-making model is proposed as a promising method of engaging patients and their families in medical decisions, especially with respect to the choice of antipsychotic and other medications.
- **FEP patients have specific pharmacotherapeutic characteristics.** FEP patients are more responsive to treatment and more sensitive to antipsychotic side effects than patients with multiple episodes (especially side effects related to dopamine blockade). Most respond to a lower antipsychotic dose than is recommended for multiple-episode patients (see page 80 on dosage of antipsychotics).

- **Reasons for relapse should be considered before switching antipsychotics.** As partial or complete nonadherence with medication is the most common reason for relapse, reasons for relapse should be considered before switching antipsychotic medications. If nonadherence has caused the relapse, reasons for this (effectiveness and tolerability) should be explored. A switch of medication is appropriate if poor tolerability has caused medication nonadherence.

- **Medication side effects should be avoided or treated early to promote response and future adherence.** All antipsychotics can cause side effects, and side effects can cause major subjective distress. As several antipsychotic side effects, such as extrapyramidal symptoms (EPS), are dose dependent and often caused by rapid titration, a low starting dose and a slow titration procedure are recommended. Early detection and treatment of side effects and early treatment adaptation are also important (see page 116). The goal is always a "minimal effective dose."

- **Short-term response predicts future response.** Antipsychotic response within the first 2–4 weeks (defined, for example, as a decrease of ≥25% in the total score on the Brief Psychiatric Rating Scale, or an increase of ≥20% in the Subjective Wellbeing under Neuroleptic Treatment scale total score predicts future responds. In cases of complete nonresponse within the first 2–4 weeks, early switching of antipsychotic medications should be considered.

- **After two unsuccessful antipsychotic trials, clozapine should be considered.** If response-confounding factors are ruled out (see section on pharmacological treatment of treatment-resistant schizophrenia [TRS]), and the patient has been treated with two different antipsychotics over a sufficient time with a sufficient dosage without success, a course of medication for TRS should be considered. Clozapine is the most appropriate antipsychotic option in TRS.

Choice of medication

The choice of medication should be determined by the drugs available in the formulary (Figure 3.2), stage of illness (eg, acute, stable), history of response and compliance, efficacy and tolerability of the available medications, effectiveness in different comorbid psychiatric disorders or suicidal behavior, and cost-effectiveness. Consideration of all these elements is required to make the right choice for a given patient, along with the considerations in the text box below. Figure 3.3 summarizes the advantages and disadvantages associated with some of the formulations of antipsychotics (for comparisons between different SGA long-acting injections [LAIs], see Figure 2.19).

Choosing medication in acute schizophrenia

- **First- and second-generation antipsychotics are not homogeneous groups of medications.** Antipsychotics within these groups are approved for different indications, have varying pharmacokinetic profiles, are available in different formulations, and have side-effect profiles of varying prevalences and intensities. Given the above factors, an antipsychotic should be chosen based on patient preference and demonstrated effectiveness for specific symptoms or syndromes and possible comorbid psychiatric conditions (eg, substance abuse disorder or major depression).
- **Currently, most guidelines recommend SGAs as first-choice treatment in patients with acute schizophrenia.** SGAs are especially preferred in patients who:
  - are antipsychotic naïve because of their high sensitivity for the occurrence of EPS;
  - have high EPS sensitivity and early stage or already existing tardive dyskinesia;
  - have primary negative symptoms (possibly in combination with an antidepressant);
  - have cognitive dysfunction (SGAs are associated with an improvement in cognitive function, although they often do not fully normalize these deficits);

Approved labeling, available formulations, and dosage strengths of commonly used first- and second-generation oral antipsychotics

Antipsychotic	Approved for	Tablet/capsule (mg)	Liquid	Short-acting intramuscular	Orally disintegrated (mg)	Long-acting injectable (mg)
Second-generation antipsychotic						
Amisulpride	S	50, 200, 400		Yes		
Aripiprazole	S, ABE, MTBD	2, 5, 10, 15, 20, 30	Yes	Yes	10, 15, 20, 30	
Asenapine	S, ABE				5, 10	
Clozapine	S	25, 100			25, 100	
Olanzapine	S, ABE, ABD, MTBD	2.5, 5, 7.5, 10, 15, 20		Yes	5, 10, 15, 20	
Paliperidone XR	S	3, 6, 9				
Quetiapine IR	S, ABE, ABD	25, 50, 100, 200, 300, 400				
Quetiapine XR	S, ABE, ABD	50, 200, 300, 400				
Risperidone	S, ABE	0.25, 0.5, 1, 2, 4	Yes		0.5, 1, 2, 3, 4	25, 37.5, 50
Ziprasidone	S, ABE	20, 40, 60, 80 (capsules)	Yes	Yes		
First-generation antipsychotic						
Chlorpromazine		10, 25, 50, 100, 200	Yes	Yes	20, 75, 150	
Haloperidol		0.5, 1, 2, 5, 10, 20	Yes	Yes		50, 100
Perphenazine		2, 4, 9, 16	Yes	Yes		100

Figure 3.2 Approved labeling, available formulations, and dosage strengths of commonly used first- and second-generation oral antipsychotics. ABD, acute bipolar depression; ABE, acute bipolar manic/mixed episodes; IR, immediate release; MTBD, maintenance treatment of bipolar disorder; S, schizophrenia; XR, extended release. Adapted from Weiden et al [6].

	Advantages	Disadvantages
Depot antipsychotics compared with oral antipsychotics	• Less frequent administration • Certainty of medication delivery, especially by overcoming covert nonadherence • Reduced fluctuations in serum concentration (avoidance of first-pass metabolism), resulting in reduction of metabolites, a decreased risk of drug interactions, and reduced dosage with fewer side effects • Reduced risk of accidental or deliberate overdose • Enriched interaction between patient and treatment team, with concomitant increase in opportunities for psychosocial support	• Delayed disappearance of distressing side effects after discontinuation of medication • Occasionally local tissue reactions at injection site
Risperidone long-acting injection compared with depot formulation first-generation antipsychotics	• Avoidance of "early peak phenomenon" with its increased risk of extrapyramidal symptoms • Avoidance of accumulation in the body with its delayed washout period if medication is discontinued	• Interaction with fluoxetine and paroxetine • Delayed onset of antipsychotic action because of gradual hydrolysis • Must be given every 2 weeks instead of monthly injections with haloperidol decanoate

Figure 3.3 Advantages and disadvantages of different formulations of antipsychotics.
Adapted from Lambert [7].

- have comorbid psychiatric conditions, especially given that SGAs have shown effectiveness as an add-on therapy in several psychiatric disorders, which are frequent in schizophrenia; and
- have already shown a poor response or experienced unacceptable side effects under first-generation antipsychotics (FGAs).

• **Patients who can be treated with FGAs are those who:**

- are currently responding well to FGAs and have no EPS, akathisia or tardive dyskinesia; and
- have a history of responding better to FGAs than to SGAs. In such cases, the lowest dose of a high-potency antipsychotic drug is usually the best choice. Thus, haloperidol 2–10 mg/day or its equivalent is effective and reasonably well tolerated in

most patients. The lowest dose is usually not effective in more chronic patients but may suffice in some FEP patients. High doses are likely to cause severe EPS. The main disadvantage of the FGAs besides EPS and the risk of tardive dyskinesia, is their lack of effect on cognition and negative symptoms.

- **Choices within each of the SGAs and FGAs classes can be additionally made on a variety of dimensions,** the most important being: formulation, cost, need for titration, effect on weight gain, lipids and risk for diabetes, EPS liability, prolactin elevations, mechanism of action, and full side-effect profile.

- **In patients with confirmed TRS, clozapine has repeatedly shown the best effectiveness.** However, as 40–70% of patients on clozapine are not free of symptoms, subsequent augmentation therapy or antipsychotic combination therapy could be necessary (see section on TRS, page 101).

- **In the acute phase, many patients require additional treatment with benzodiazepines,** such as for managing agitation (eg, diazepam), anxiety (eg, lorazepam) or sleep disturbance (eg, oxazepam). Treatment with benzodiazepines should be used with caution in patients with comorbid substance abuse disorder.

- **For the treatment of behavioral emergencies, there are several short-acting injectable antipsychotic formulations** These formulations should be applied according to guidelines for behavioral emergencies in schizophrenia (see section on the treatment of behavioral emergencies, page 93).

- **With the approval of the first SGA LAIs, prescribing practice for depot antipsychotics has changed.** Risperidone LAI (RLAI) is the first second-generation depot antipsychotic. It is enclosed in "microspheres," which are injected into the body, and slowly dissolve, releasing a constant amount of the risperidone medication. Depot antipsychotics have several advantages compared with oral antipsychotics, and some disadvantages, as does RLAI compared with conventional depot antipsychotics.

Dosage of antipsychotics

Despite years of clinical and research experience, definitive dose–response curves do not exist for antipsychotic drugs. Figure 3.4 summarizes dosage recommendations for various oral FGAs and SGAs.

Determining the dosage for antipsychotics

- **The minimal effective dose (best effectiveness and side-effect ratio) should be chosen.** Lower doses are generally recommended in: (1) FEP patients, who tend to be more responsive to treatment and more sensitive to side effects; (2) elderly people, who may metabolize antipsychotic drugs at substantially lower rates and may also be more sensitive to side effects; and (3) women, who often require lower overall antipsychotic dosages and are sensitive to prolactin-related side effects.

- **The optimal dose range for FGAs is between 300 mg and 800 mg chlorpromazine equivalents per day** (6–16 mg haloperidol equivalents per day). There are no significant advantages to using dosages of haloperidol >10–20 mg/day for acute treatment; indeed, dosages of 20 mg may be associated with a substantial number of adverse neurologic effects if prophylactic antiparkinsonian medication is not also given.

- **The dose recommendations for SGAs in clinical practice are consistent with their respective summaries of product information, with some exceptions:**
  - Studies of the starting dose of quetiapine immediate release (IR; 200–300 mg/day) and ziprasidone (80 mg/day) have shown successful initiation of treatment with higher than the approved initial dose.
  - Studies of quetiapine IR have found that a titration scheme other than the licensed one was comparably well tolerated (200 mg → 400 mg → 600 mg → 800 mg from day 1 to day 4). Whether it is more effective than the recommended one is still unclear.

Recommended dosages of selected oral first- and second-generation antipsychotics in the acute treatment of schizophrenia

Antipsychotic	Usual starting dosage (mg/day)	Dose interval*	Target dose first episode (mg/day)	Target dose multiple episodes (mg/day)	Maximal dosage (mg/day)[†]	Recommended plasma level (c)
Second-generation antipsychotic						
Amisulpride	200	1–2	100–300	400–800	1200	100–400
Aripiprazole	10–15	1	5–15	15–30	30	150–250
Asenapine	5–10	2	5–15	10–20	20	NA
Clozapine[‡]	25	2–4	100–250	200–450	900	350–600
Olanzapine	5–10	1	5–15	5–20	20[†]	20–80
Paliperidone[†]	6	1	3–6	3–9	12[†]	NA
Quetiapine IR or XR	50–300	IR: 2, XR: 1	300–600	400–750	750[†]	70–170
Risperidone	2	1–2	1–4	3–6	6	20–60
Ziprasidone	40–80	2	40–80	80–160	160[†]	50–120
Zotepine	25–50	2–4	50–150	75–150	450	12–120
First-generation antipsychotic						
Chlorpromazine	50–150	2–4	300–500	300–1000	1000	30–300
Fluphenazine	0.4–10	2–3	2.4–10	10–20	20–40	0.5–2
Haloperidol	1–10	1–2	1–4	3–15	100	5–17
Perphenazine	4–24	1–3	6–36	12–42	56	0.6–2.4

Figure 3.4 Recommended dosages of selected oral first- and second-generation antipsychotics in the acute treatment of schizophrenia. *Recommended distribution of the daily total dose: one time point = 1, two time points = 2, etc.; if applicable, higher than recommended doses have to be distributed on several time points. [†]Highest approved dose; there are positive experiences with higher than approved doses in special populations, especially with some second-generation antipsychotics. [‡]Clozapine is usually not indicated in first-episode psychosis. IR, immediate release; XR, extended release. Adapted from Lambert [7].

> – Several case reports suggest that a number of SGAs possibly have some positive effects in doses above the licensed range. However, robust controlled data (eg, on quetiapine) suggest that the standard dose range is appropriate for clinical use in most cases.

Therapeutic drug monitoring

It is known that therapeutic drug monitoring (TDM) increases the likelihood of response and reduces the risk of antipsychotic side effects for some antipsychotics. TDM should be part of standard care for these medications. Within the FGA group, this is known for haloperidol, perphenazine, and fluphenazine; in the SGA group, for clozapine, olanzapine, and risperidone (Figure 3.5). TDM is important in patients treated with TRS who have shown a higher response rate for plasma levels >350 ng/mL (8–38% at <350 ng/mL vs 50–75% at >350 ng/mL) [8,9].

There are also several other indications for TDM:

- when patients fail to respond to what is usually an adequate dose;
- when it is difficult to discriminate drug side effects from symptoms, such as agitation or negative impairments (eg, a high blood level might be associated with increased adverse effects);
- when antipsychotic drugs are combined with other drugs that may affect their pharmacokinetics (drug–drug interactions), such as fluvoxamine, fluoxetine, or carbamazepine;
- in very young children, elderly people, and patients who are medically compromised, in whom the pharmacokinetics of antipsychotics may be significantly altered (eg, patients with renal and/or liver insufficiency or cardiovascular disease [CVD]);
- when noncompliance or poor compliance is suspected or when compliance is imposed by the legal system; and
- for monitoring of medications with compulsive TDM for safety reasons (eg, lithium).

Therapeutic drug monitoring for different antipsychotics

Antipsychotic	Recommended plasma levels (ng/mL)*	Recommendations for the use of TDM†
Second-generation antipsychotic		
Amisulpride	100–400	3
Aripiprazole	150–250	4
Asenapine	3–5	4
Clozapine	350–600	1
Olanzapine	20–80	1
Paliperidone	?	?
Quetiapine IR	70–170	3
Quetiapine XR	?	?
Risperidone	20–60	2
Ziprasidone	50–120	4
Zotepine	12–120	3
First-generation antipsychotic		
Chlorpromazine	30–300	2
Fluphenazine	0.5–2	1
Flupenthixol	>2	2
Haloperidol	5–17	1
Perazine	100–230	2
Perphenazine	0.6–2.4	2
Zuclopenthixol	4–50	3

Figure 3.5 Therapeutic drug monitoring for different antipsychotics. *Recommended plasma levels are medication concentrations in serum or plasma within the steady state with the highest chance of antipsychotic response. †The graduation is the estimation for the usefulness of TDM for dosage optimization: (1) highly recommended: several studies support the usefulness of TDM; (2) recommended: at least one prospective study has shown a relationship between plasma concentration and antipsychotic response and there are reports about intoxications within concentrations above the normal range; (3) useful: retrospective studies and single case reports make it plausible that there is a relation between plasma concentration and antipsychotic response; (4) possibly useful: pharmacokinetic studies can be used to show plasma concentrations within therapeutic effective dosages; (5) not recommended: the use of TDM in pharmacological studies is not useful. IR, immediate release; TDM, therapeutic drug monitoring; XR, extended release. Adapted from Lambert [7].

Antipsychotic treatment algorithm for acute schizophrenia

Algorithms for treatment of schizophrenia are helpful tools for understanding the course and order of subsequent intervention steps. Figure 3.6 presents an algorithm for the treatment of acute schizophrenia.

Starting with a second-generation antipsychotic

In nonemergency acute schizophrenia, most patients should start antipsychotic treatment with an SGA. At this time, seven different SGAs are available, along with paliperidone and quetiapine extended-release formulations. Choice of medication depends on various factors, which have been described above and are shown in Figure 3.6. In patients with psychotic relapse, the assessment of potential reasons for relapse is the main requirement for an adequate choice of medication. In most, the reason for relapse is partial or full nonadherence with medication. Therefore, simply choosing a new antipsychotic is probably not the optimal approach because nonadherence is markedly influenced by other factors.

Starting with monotherapy

It should be emphasized that treatment should start with a single antipsychotic drug, and the choice should be based on tolerability, efficacy, and cost-effectiveness. Patients should receive an adequate trial without casual addition of a second antipsychotic drug for the duration of that trial, which can then be terminated if there is lack of efficacy or tolerability. Furthermore, the evidence to support the concurrent use of a mood stabilizer or antidepressant during the initial stages of treatment is minimal, so clinicians should be cautious in starting treatment with both an antipsychotic and one or both of these other drug types.

Starting dose, titration scheme, and target dose

The starting dose, titration, and target dose depend on several factors:

- The target dose for a specific antipsychotic depends on the optimal dose range separated into antipsychotic-naïve and antipsychotic-adjusted patients.
- Antipsychotic-naïve patients should generally start on a lower dose, and their target dose is lower compared with antipsychotic-adjusted multiple-episode patients (a 24- to 48-hour antipsychotic-free interval should be considered if indicated).
- Higher starting doses, accelerated titration schemes, and higher target doses are recommended in very acute patients.

Algorithm for the treatment of acute schizophrenia

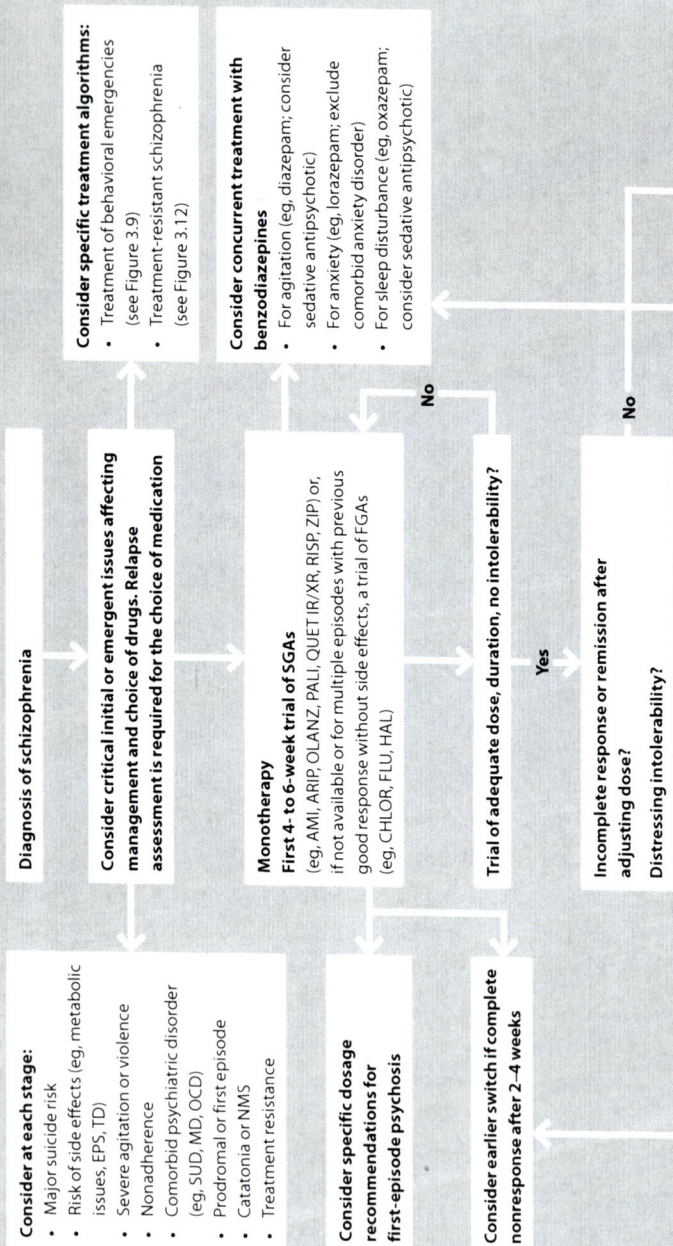

Consider at each stage:
- Major suicide risk
- Risk of side effects (eg, metabolic issues, EPS, TD)
- Severe agitation or violence
- Nonadherence
- Comorbid psychiatric disorder (eg, SUD, MD, OCD)
- Prodromal or first episode
- Catatonia or NMS
- Treatment resistance

Consider specific dosage recommendations for first-episode psychosis

Consider earlier switch if complete nonresponse after 2–4 weeks

Diagnosis of schizophrenia

↓

Consider critical initial or emergent issues affecting management and choice of drugs. Relapse assessment is required for the choice of medication

↓

Monotherapy
First 4- to 6-week trial of SGAs
(eg, AMI, ARIP, OLANZ, PALI, QUET IR/XR, RISP, ZIP) or, if not available or for multiple episodes with previous good response without side effects, a trial of FGAs (eg, CHLOR, FLU, HAL)

↓

Trial of adequate dose, duration, no intolerability?

— Yes →

Incomplete response or remission after adjusting dose?
Distressing intolerability?

— No →

Consider specific treatment algorithms:
- Treatment of behavioral emergencies (see Figure 3.9)
- Treatment-resistant schizophrenia (see Figure 3.12)

Consider concurrent treatment with benzodiazepines
- For agitation (eg, diazepam; consider sedative antipsychotic)
- For anxiety (eg, lorazepam; exclude comorbid anxiety disorder)
- For sleep disturbance (eg, oxazepam; consider sedative antipsychotic)

No →

No →

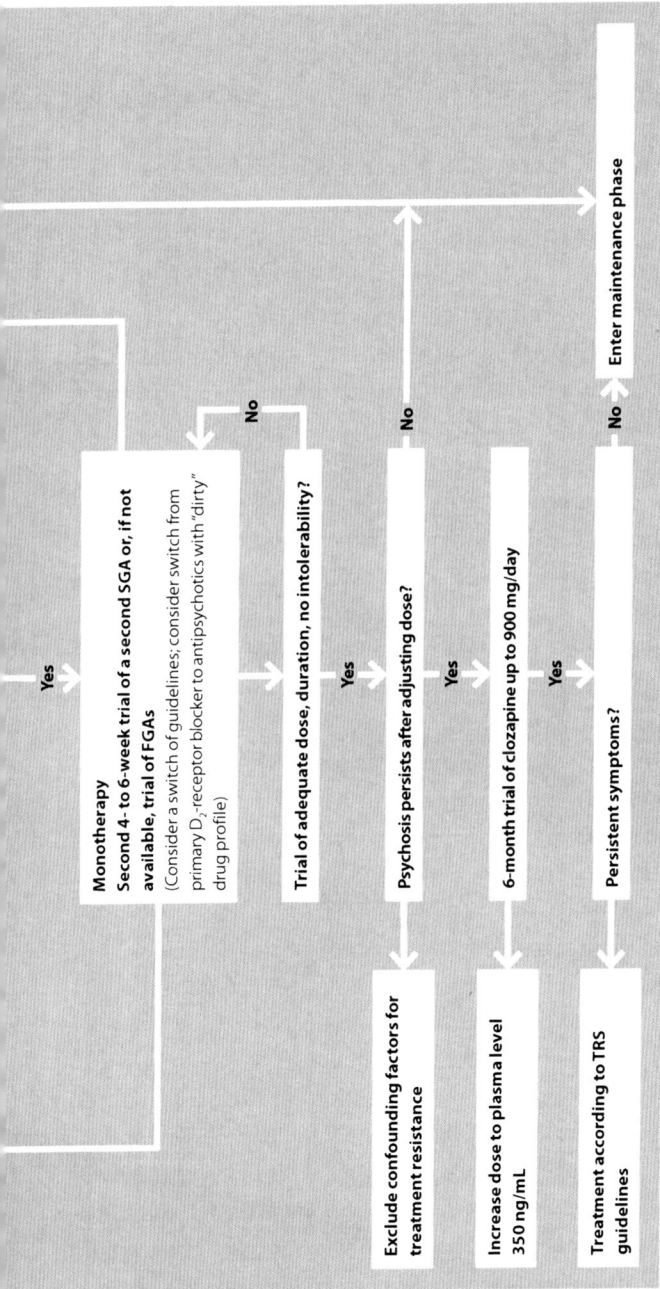

Figure 3.6 Algorithm for the treatment of acute schizophrenia. AMI, amisulpride; ARIP, aripiprazole; CHLOR, chlorpromazine; CLOZ, clozapine; D, dopamine; EPS, extrapyramidal symptoms; FGA, first-generation antipsychotic; FLU, fluphenazine; HAL, haloperidol; IR, immediate release; MD, manic depression; NMS, neuroleptic malignant syndrome; OCD, obsessive–compulsive disorder; OLANZ, olanzapine; PALI, paliperidone; QUET, quetiapine; RISP, risperidone; SGA, second-generation antipsychotic; SUD, substance use disorder; TD, tardive dyskinesia; TRS, treatment-resistant schizophrenia; XR, extended release; zip, ziprasidone. Adapted from the International Psychopharmacology Algorithm Project [10].

- Antipsychotics in extended-release formulations can be immediately started at an effective dose.
- For the treatment of primary negative symptoms (deficit syndrome) a lower target dose is recommended.
- The risk of side effects related to a specific antipsychotic and to individual risk factors should finally guide the starting dose, titration scheme, and target dose.

Factors determining antipsychotic response

Response can be partial or full, or there can be complete nonresponse, depending on several factors. Some of these factors are not related to a specific antipsychotic, including long DUP, persistent comorbid substance abuse, and a low premorbid functioning level. Factors related to antipsychotics include an adequate dose and an adequate duration of treatment. At present, guidelines recommend waiting for 4–6 weeks before considering a patient with schizophrenia to be a nonresponder and before switching antipsychotics. However, several study results have questioned this clinical practice. Early response studies have shown that:

- the major psychopathological improvement occurs within the first week;
- no or only minimal improvement in the first 2 weeks predicts nonresponse after 4–6 weeks; and
- the symptomatic improvement within the first 4 weeks is significantly higher than the additional change during the following year.

Overall, these results have led to questioning of the commonly held "delayed-onset" hypothesis of antipsychotic drugs. Nevertheless, a trial of a single antipsychotic should generally last 2–6 weeks, with at least 2–4 weeks on a dose within the therapeutic range.

A failed trial is one in which the medication dose and duration were adequate and no concomitant medication might be expected to interfere with efficacy, but in which clinical response in core outcome measures, particularly control of positive symptoms, was inadequate and had plateaued at an inadequate level. A trial terminated for lack of tolerability before it meets these criteria should not be considered an adequate trial.

Switching antipsychotics

The decision to switch an antipsychotic can be based on insufficient efficacy, unacceptable tolerability, or other reasons (eg, patient's wish). Some strategies for switching antipsychotics should be taken into account (Figure 3.7).

Guidelines for switching antipsychotics

- Before considering switching, the dose of the current treatment should be optimized to give it an adequate trial. Some side effects decrease over time (eg, sedation, hypotension) and it is worth waiting for adaptation. Comorbid symptoms/disorders should be treated adequately before a switch is made. It should be noted that a switch from clozapine to another antipsychotic is often unsuccessful; in such instances, assisting patients to cope with side effects is worthwhile.
- The decision to switch is mainly based on an efficacy and tolerability ratio, with realistic expectations.
- When deciding whether to switch, drug efficacy, receptor profile, tolerability and safety should be considered, as well as variables regarding the patient, illness, and patient's environment.
- Psychoeducation should be provided and the patient and family should be involved in the decision-making process.
- Switching should be done in a crossover procedure; with few exceptions; abrupt switching is neither advisable nor necessary. Crossover has two main advantages: (1) lower relapse risk and (2) reduced likelihood of physical and mental withdrawal reactions.
- Switch should be slower in females and older patients.
- There are three different crossover procedures: (1) taper switch; (2) cross-taper switch; and (3) plateau cross-taper switch.
- For patients with unacceptable side effects procedures (1) and (2) are recommended; for patients with insufficiently treated symptoms (3) is recommended. It should be noted that procedure (3) has a greater risk of keeping patients on polyantipsychotic treatment because of enhanced efficacy during the switch.

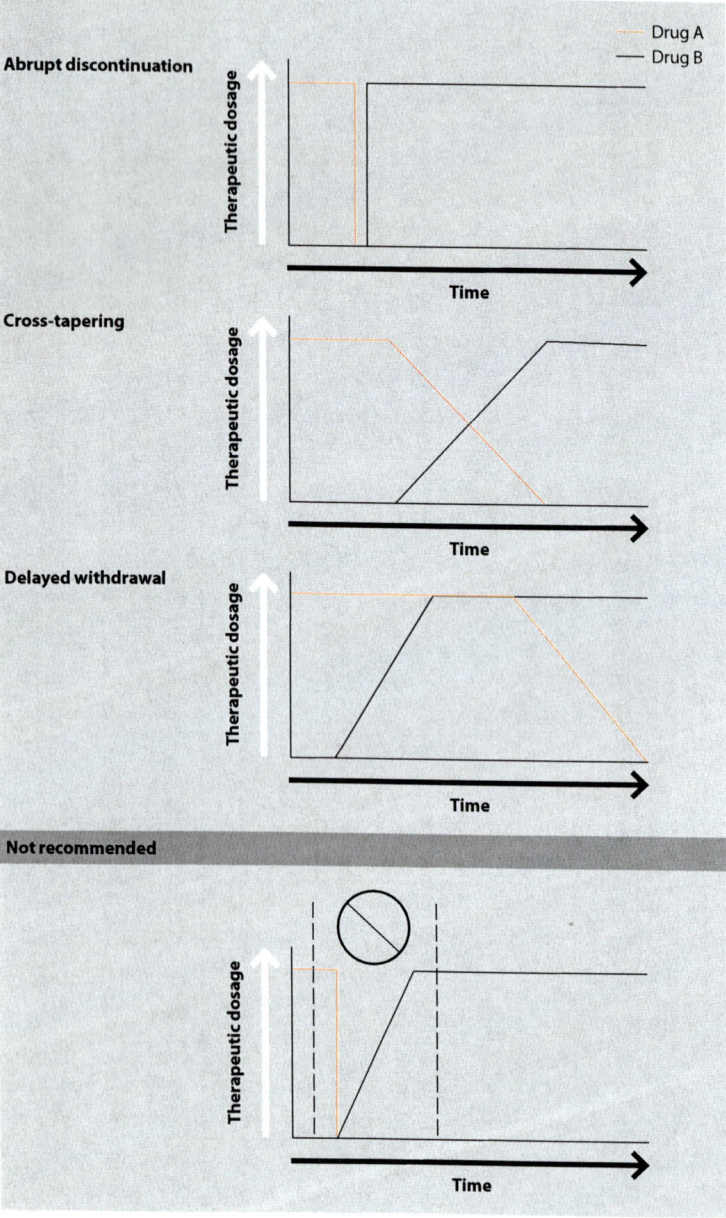

Figure 3.7 Antipsychotic switching strategies. Adapted from Lambert [7].

- If changes are not needed, other medications should not be changed during the switching period.
- Vigilance for emerging side effects or withdrawal symptoms, and appropriate treatment, are required (add respective medication and continue for at least 2 weeks after the side effects disappear).
- Physicians should be available to deal with potential problems.

There are no clear data to indicate which antipsychotic should be tried when an adequate trial of another antipsychotic fails to control positive symptoms. Before turning to clozapine, most guidelines recommend a second monotherapy trial with an SGA other than clozapine if patients have persistent psychotic symptoms. The choice of the second drug depends upon the first drug and reasons that may have contributed to the treatment failure. In addition, some experts recommend a switch from primary dopamine D_2-receptor blocker (eg, risperidone or amisulpride) to antipsychotics with a "dirty" drug profile (multireceptor antipsychotics, such as quetiapine or olanzapine) and vice versa.

Determining whether there is treatment resistance

Approximately 30% of patients might be expected to have an unsatisfactory response to two trials of SGAs or FGAs if the inadequate response is defined as persistence of moderate-to-severe delusions, hallucinations, and disorganized thinking [11,12]. Patients should also be considered treatment resistant if they have severe negative symptoms, suicidal thoughts, or aggressive behavior on a chronic basis despite the control of positive symptoms. Clinical evidence suggests that treatment with clozapine is indicated for the patient with schizophrenia who has failed two trials with other antipsychotic drugs, regardless of class. For further treatment recommendations on the pharmacological management of TRS see page 101.

Treatment of behavioral emergencies

During an acute psychotic episode of schizophrenia, some patients become behaviorally disturbed and may need emergency pharmacological (and psychological) interventions. In the USA, 21% of all behavioral emergencies are due to agitation in schizophrenia [13]. On admission to hospital, 14% of all patients with schizophrenia show aggressive behavior; and 8–10% have to be physically restrained at least once in their life [14]. There is a variety of preventive strategies to decrease the incidence and severity of behavioral emergencies in schizophrenia:

- education and community awareness about schizophrenia;
- environment adaptation (intensive care area in the acute ward);
- implementation of action by an assertive community treatment team, with the goal of early detection of deterioration, relapse, and behavioral emergencies;
- aggression management training and education for staff;
- early detection of behavioral emergencies during inpatient treatment (ie, assessment of risk factors and regular assessment of behavioral disturbances in patients at risk);
- use of interpreters for patients who have language difficulties; and
- early treatment of low levels of agitation and sleep disturbances.

There are various risk factors for agitation in schizophrenia (Figure 3.8), and diagnostic tests may be an important adjunct to the history and physical examination of the agitated schizophrenic patient. Treatable medical conditions should be ruled out. However, most commonly,

Risk factors for agitation in schizophrenia

- Male gender
- Medication nonadherence
- Severe psychopathology, especially delusions and hallucinations
- Disorganized subtype of schizophrenia
- Comorbid personality disorder or traits (especially antisocial or borderline)
- Comorbid substance abuse disorder
- Current drug and/or alcohol intoxication
- Admission against will
- History of aggressive behavior
- Language difficulties
- Low IQ
- Hearing problems

Figure 3.8 Risk factors for agitation in schizophrenia. Adapted from Allen et al [14].

agitation results from nonadherence to maintenance therapy and disease progression. The goal of emergency management is to assure safety for patients and staff alike, and to resolve the situation without harm and traumatic experiences.

Nonpharmacological interventions in behavioral emergencies

There are various possible nonpharmacological interventions, such as placing the patient in a quiet nonthreatening environment (eg, intensive care area), reduction of external noise and other stimuli, behavioral management (ie, granting privileges for appropriate behavior), close observation, calm conversation, and active listening. The clinician should avoid unprepared confrontations; where possible, the patient's key clinician should establish the patient's concerns and attempt to resolve conflict.

Pharmacological interventions in behavioral emergencies

Oral antipsychotics as first-line therapy

Before resorting to the emergency use of acute intramuscular agents, the first-line pharmacotherapeutic intervention is to convince the patient to accept oral antipsychotic preparations (Figure 3.9). There are two possibilities:

1. Use of antipsychotic monotherapy – an emergency high dose of an atypical antipsychotic at first (day 1) and an emergency maintenance dose (days 2–5) – has been found to be effective.
2. Use of an antipsychotic and benzodiazepine combination (eg, risperidone [liquid] plus lorazepam [orally dissolving tablet]) has been found to be as effective as haloperidol (intramuscular) plus lorazepam (orally dissolving tablet).

In many patients, this step is sufficient to resolve the crisis, although it should be noted that the use of adjunctive benzodiazepines is restricted or contraindicated in older patients with schizophrenia or if drug or alcohol intoxication has caused the emergency. If the patient refuses medication, the next step is "show of force." In this, a larger group of staff tries to convince the patient to accept oral medication by explaining that parenteral medication will be necessary if he or she will not accept oral medication.

Treatment algorithm for behavioral emergencies in acute schizophrenia

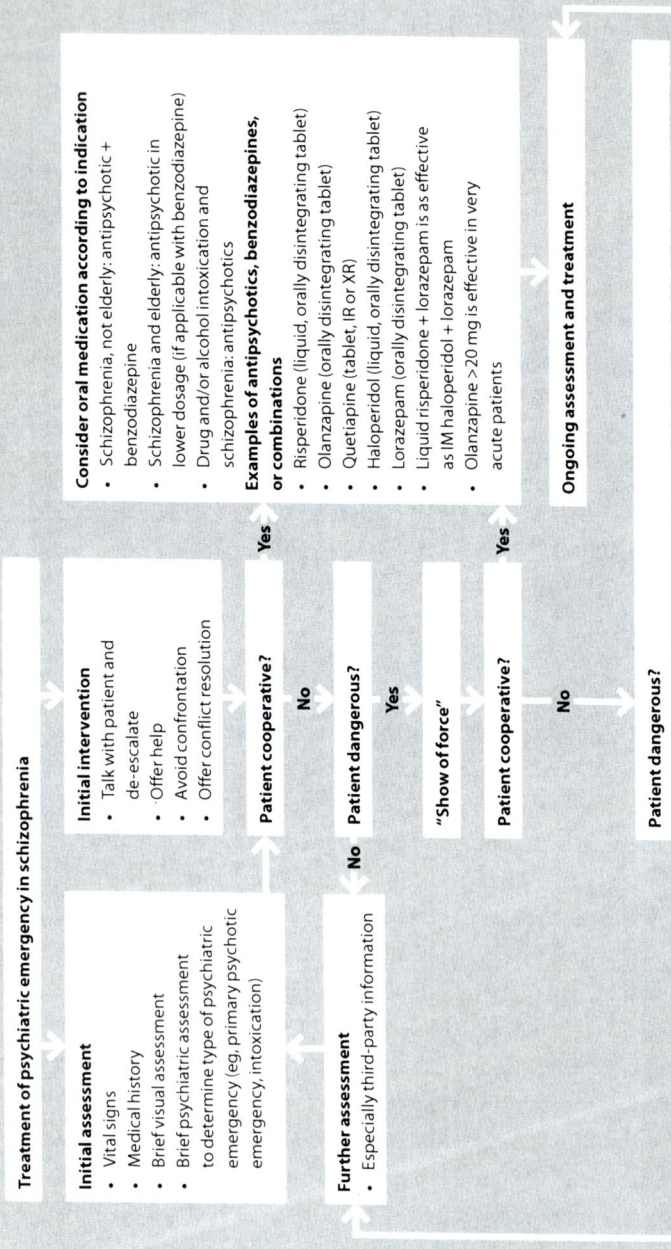

Treatment of psychiatric emergency in schizophrenia

Initial assessment
- Vital signs
- Medical history
- Brief visual assessment
- Brief psychiatric assessment to determine type of psychiatric emergency (eg, primary psychotic emergency, intoxication)

Further assessment
- Especially third-party information

Initial intervention
- Talk with patient and de-escalate
- Offer help
- Avoid confrontation
- Offer conflict resolution

Patient cooperative?

No / Yes

Patient dangerous?

No / Yes

"Show of force"

Patient cooperative?

No / Yes

Patient dangerous?

Consider oral medication according to indication
- Schizophrenia, not elderly: antipsychotic + benzodiazepine
- Schizophrenia and elderly: antipsychotic in lower dosage (if applicable with benzodiazepine)
- Drug and/or alcohol intoxication and schizophrenia: antipsychotics

Examples of antipsychotics, benzodiazepines, or combinations
- Risperidone (liquid, orally disintegrating tablet)
- Olanzapine (orally disintegrating tablet)
- Quetiapine (tablet, IR or XR)
- Haloperidol (liquid, orally disintegrating tablet)
- Lorazepam (orally disintegrating tablet)
- Liquid risperidone + lorazepam is as effective as IM haloperidol + lorazepam
- Olanzapine >20 mg is effective in very acute patients

Ongoing assessment and treatment

Establish possible cause

Psychiatric cause

No

Somatic cause

Yes

Parenteral medication with or without physical restraint
- Ensure safety for patients and staff
- Regular monitoring of vital signs and psychiatric state

Consider parenteral medication according to indication
- Ziprasidone 20 mg IM*
- Olanzapine 10 mg IM†
- Haloperidol 5 mg IM‡ + lorazepam 2 mg IM‡
- Lorazepam 2 mg IM†
- Haloperidol 10 mg IM‡
- Haloperidol 2 mg IM‡
- Olanzapine 5 mg IM†
- Haloperidol 5–10 mg IM‡
- Ziprasidone 20 mg IM*

Schizophrenia, not elderly

Schizophrenia and elderly

Drug and/or alcohol intoxication

Debriefing for patient and staff, if applicable also for others (eg, relatives). Patient should be in remission of acute agitation

Patient cooperative?

Yes

No

Reconsider diagnosis and cause

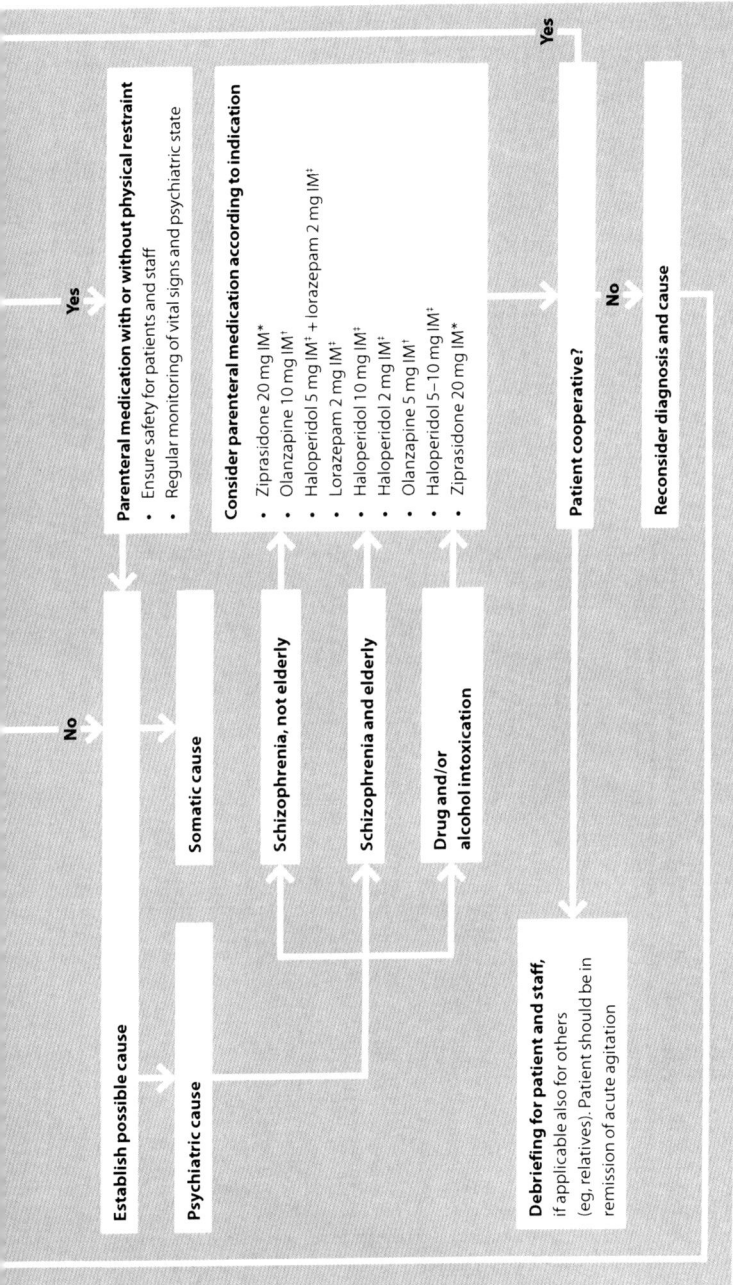

Figure 3.9 Treatment algorithm for behavioral emergencies in acute schizophrenia. *Do not use in case of prolonged QTc interval; †not for use together with benzodiazepines; ‡also in intravenous form. IM, intramuscular; IR, immediate release; XR, extended release. Adapted from Allen et al [14].

Intramuscular antipsychotics as second-line pharmacotherapy
If the patient still refuses medication, or if a rapid response is needed due
to violent behavior or other disturbances, parenteral medication (intramuscular injection) will be necessary (Figure 3.10). In this situation, team
members must all ensure that they clearly and calmly communicate the
necessity of parenteral medication to the patient. Here, it is necessary
to understand that agitation usually results from psychotic anxiety and
that measures taken against the will of the patient can exacerbate this
anxiety and lead to traumatization. Therefore, such a decision should be

Recommended indications and doses of intramuscular medications for emergency treatment of schizophrenia

Medication	Approved indications	Dosage (mg)
Lorazepam IM	• Psychiatric emergency • Status epilepticus • Pre-anesthetic • Anxiety state	• 0.5–2.5 • Up to 10 mg/day • IV not more than 2 mg in one application
Haloperidol IM	• Schizophrenia • Psychotic disorders, especially paranoid • Mania and hypomania • Behavioral disturbances in mental retardation or organic brain damage • Adjunct therapy in psychomotor agitation, excitement, violent or dangerously impulsive behavior • Nausea and vomiting	0.5–7.5
Ziprasidone IM*	• Agitation • Psychotic disorders	10–20
Olanzapine IM†	• Agitation • Psychotic disorders • Bipolar disorder	10
Zuclopenthixol acuphase IM	• Agitation • Psychotic disorders • Bipolar disorder	50–150

Figure 3.10 **Recommended indications and doses of intramuscular medications for emergency treatment of schizophrenia.** *Do not use in case of prolonged QTc interval; †do not use together with benzodiazepines. EPS, extrapyramidal symptoms; IM, intramuscular; IV, intravenous; PPL, peak plasma level. Adapted from Lambert et al [15].

taken only after all alternatives have been considered and a psychiatrist has been consulted.

Short-acting intramuscular haloperidol or its equivalent are the most widely used medications for emergency treatment of schizophrenia [16]. Doses of 5 mg are usually given and may be repeated at intervals as needed [17]. The maximum total daily dose of short-acting intramuscular haloperidol should not exceed 20 mg/day [17]. For patients receiving short-acting intramuscular haloperidol, it is recommended that anticholinergics be started at the time of the first injection and continued

PPL (h)	Advantages	Disadvantages
10–20	• Treatment of concurrent alcohol withdrawal • IV application possible	• No antipsychotic effect • Respiratory depression
12–36	• Persistent antipsychotic effect • IV application possible	• EPS • Reduced epileptic threshold • No treatment of concurrent alcohol withdrawal
2.2–3.4	• Persistent antipsychotic effect • No or low risk for EPS	• QTc prolongation • No treatment of concurrent alcohol withdrawal • Less experience compared with other drug IM options
34–38	• Persistent antipsychotic effect • No or low risk for EPS	• No concurrent treatment with benzodiazepines possible • No treatment of concurrent alcohol withdrawal • Weight gain with long-term treatment • Less experience compared with other drug IM options
36	• In most cases no repeated injections necessary	• EPS • Contraindication in case of alcohol and/or drug intoxication • Severe sedation • Delayed onset of action (6–8 h after injection)

for at least 1 week. Alternative SGAs are intramuscular olanzapine and intramuscular ziprasidone. Intramuscular olanzapine is usually given in doses of 2.5–10 mg [18]; the acute dose of intramuscular ziprasidone is 10–20 mg [19]. Intramuscular ziprasidone and haloperidol have been shown to prolong QTc to the same extent. Serious cardiac adverse effects with ziprasidone appear to be fairly rare in the absence of pre-existent cardiac conduction disorders or other predisposing risk factors; no cases of torsades de pointes have been reported with intramuscular or oral ziprasidone [20].

Treatment with intramuscular SGAs might be recommended in patients with known risk of developing EPS or other situations where it is imperative to avoid EPS (eg, patients with FEP for whom possible dystonic reactions would be most distressing). Apart from short-acting SGAs, short-acting intramuscular benzodiazepines (eg, lorazepam) may be helpful as an adjunctive treatment or an alternative to intramuscular antipsychotic drugs.

In prolonged emergencies, a well-established option to avoid repeated intramuscular injections is the use of short-acting depot medications (eg, zuclopenthixol acetate [note zuclopenthixol acetate, is not approved in the US]) [21]. A disadvantage of this is the delayed onset of action (2–8 hours) [22], although patients may respond after 30–45 minutes. Zuclopenthixol acetate is effective for 24–36 hours [23]; repeated zuclo-penthixol injections within 24 hours of a previous dose are mostly not required (Figures 3.9 and 3.10). As a result of concerns about its pro-longation of the QTc interval (see page 136), intramuscular droperidol should not be a first-line option for the agitated psychotic patient [24]. It is not appropriate to start long-acting depot preparations in this setting.

After parenteral tranquillization, vital parameters should be moni-tored, including temperature, pulse, blood pressure, and respiratory rate, every 10 minutes for 1 hour, then half-hourly to hourly according to the half-life of the medication. Caution should be applied because of the risk of reduced respiratory rate, irregular or slow pulse, fall in blood pres-sure, or unconsciousness. Patients receiving high-potency conventional antipsychotics in short-acting intramuscular forms should be monitored daily for signs of acute dystonia, akathisia, or impending neuroleptic malignant syndrome (NMS). If available, electrocardiogram monitoring is also recommended. With the reduction of the severity of the situation, and growing awareness and less traumatic reactions in the patient, staff, family members or other caregivers should have a "debriefing process." All emergency steps including the debriefing process should be documented.

Pharmacological management of treatment-resistant schizophrenia

The management of patients with TRS includes early detection and pharmacological and psychosocial treatment. Early detection of TRS represents a significant clinical challenge because it is complicated by several factors:

- the multidimensional nature of TRS;
- the absence of distinct categories along the continuous spectrum from treatment response to complete nonresponse; and
- the lack of generally valid predictors for TRS.

Early identification is a major objective because pharmacological and psychological interventions for refractory patients differ from those for nonrefractory patients. The possibility of TRS should be considered right from the start of treatment. This recommendation, especially evident for patients who fulfill the diagnostic criterion of the *Diagnostic and Statistical Manual of Mental Disorders, 4th Edition* of 6-month duration of psychotic symptoms at initial presentation, is mainly based on the following research results:

- Several of the risk factors for TRS are already evident at initial presentation.
- Patient presents with factors related to TRS (Figure 3.11), such as structural brain abnormalities, long duration of untreated psychosis, or poor premorbid functioning, some of which are not treatable by this stage. As such, patients with certain risk factors have to be monitored for TRS early in treatment.
- Response in the first 3–6 months after start of initial antipsychotic treatment is highly predictive for subsequent TRS [11,12].
- With each relapse, there is a greater risk for secondary TRS.

Patients with TRS require specific pharmacological interventions, best applied according to a TRS treatment algorithm. Pharmacological treatment of TRS is a difficult task because resistance to treatment can occur in various phenomenological domains including symptoms, psychosocial functioning, and quality of life, and pharmacological and psychosocial interventions for each of these domains can differ markedly (Figure 3.11). However, in most cases treatment resistance affects many of these domains simultaneously. Pharmacological management of TRS can be conducted in four stages, as follows.

Stage 1
At first, the phenomenological domain affected by treatment resistance must be identified (see Figure 3.11). However, it is rare that only one domain is affected, and in most cases there are typical domain combinations affected by TRS:
- chronic delusions and concurrent social and behavioral deviations, such as recurrent aggression and hostility;
- chronic acoustic hallucinations with impaired social functioning; and
- chronic negative symptoms with concurrent cognitive deficits and social withdrawal and vocational deficits.

In stage 1, the clinician must also ensure that the patient truly meets the criteria for TRS. There are a variety of confounding factors that have to be explored and excluded before TRS is diagnosed (Figure 3.12). These are clinical factors that simulate resistance even when the patient is not truly resistant to treatment. Some of the most common and important factors are insufficient previous pharmacological interventions, repeated medication nonadherence, persistent substance abuse, and insufficient previous psychosocial treatment. At this stage it is therefore necessary to review risk factors for TRS, the type and success of previous interventions, and the respective course of illness.

The most common scenario is that the patient already had several TRS risk factors at initial presentation (eg, long DUP, poor premorbid functioning, lack of insight), was already responding poorly to the first treatment, and was repeatedly nonadhering to medication with subsequent relapse and illness progression. Review of the course of illness and treatment history should, at the same time, guide the optimization

Factors related to treatment-resistant schizophrenia

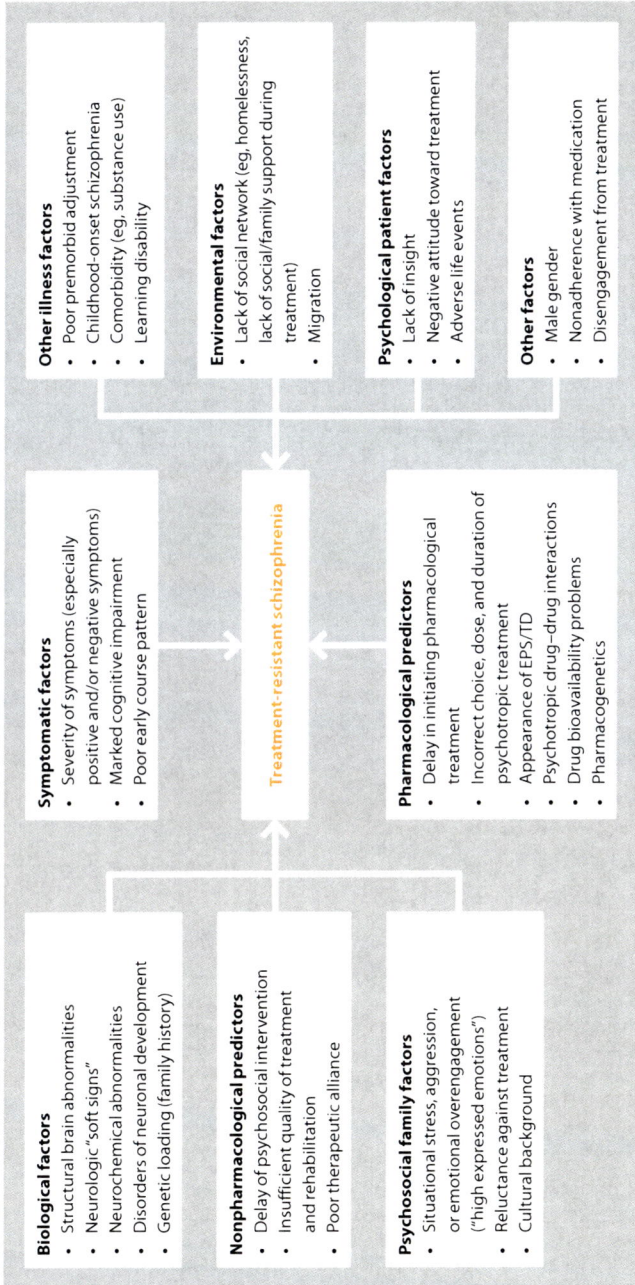

Biological factors
- Structural brain abnormalities
- Neurologic "soft signs"
- Neurochemical abnormalities
- Disorders of neuronal development
- Genetic loading (family history)

Nonpharmacological predictors
- Delay of psychosocial intervention
- Insufficient quality of treatment and rehabilitation
- Poor therapeutic alliance

Psychosocial family factors
- Situational stress, aggression, or emotional overengagement ("high expressed emotions")
- Reluctance against treatment
- Cultural background

Symptomatic factors
- Severity of symptoms (especially positive and/or negative symptoms)
- Marked cognitive impairment
- Poor early course pattern

Treatment-resistant schizophrenia

Pharmacological predictors
- Delay in initiating pharmacological treatment
- Incorrect choice, dose, and duration of psychotropic treatment
- Appearance of EPS/TD
- Psychotropic drug–drug interactions
- Drug bioavailability problems
- Pharmacogenetics

Other illness factors
- Poor premorbid adjustment
- Childhood-onset schizophrenia
- Comorbidity (eg, substance use)
- Learning disability

Environmental factors
- Lack of social network (eg, homelessness, lack of social/family support during treatment)
- Migration

Psychological patient factors
- Lack of insight
- Negative attitude toward treatment
- Adverse life events

Other factors
- Male gender
- Nonadherence with medication
- Disengagement from treatment

Figure 3.11 Factors related to treatment-resistant schizophrenia. EPS, extrapyramidal symptoms; TD, tardive dyskinesia. Adapted from Huber et al [11] and Lambert et al [12].

Pharmacotherapeutic algorithm for treatment-resistant schizophrenia

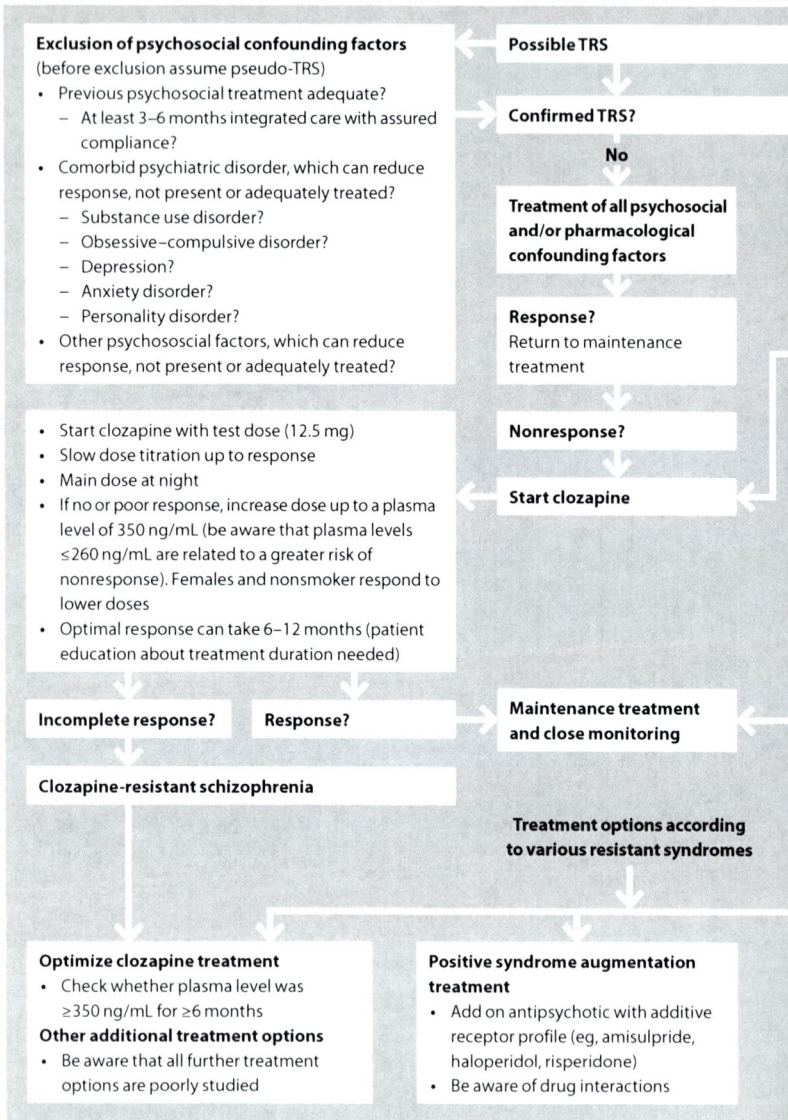

Exclusion of psychosocial confounding factors
(before exclusion assume pseudo-TRS)
- Previous psychosocial treatment adequate?
  - At least 3–6 months integrated care with assured compliance?
- Comorbid psychiatric disorder, which can reduce response, not present or adequately treated?
  - Substance use disorder?
  - Obsessive–compulsive disorder?
  - Depression?
  - Anxiety disorder?
  - Personality disorder?
- Other psychososcial factors, which can reduce response, not present or adequately treated?

Possible TRS

Confirmed TRS?

No

Treatment of all psychosocial and/or pharmacological confounding factors

Response?
Return to maintenance treatment

- Start clozapine with test dose (12.5 mg)
- Slow dose titration up to response
- Main dose at night
- If no or poor response, increase dose up to a plasma level of 350 ng/mL (be aware that plasma levels ≤260 ng/mL are related to a greater risk of nonresponse). Females and nonsmoker respond to lower doses
- Optimal response can take 6–12 months (patient education about treatment duration needed)

Nonresponse?

Start clozapine

Incomplete response?   **Response?**

Maintenance treatment and close monitoring

Clozapine-resistant schizophrenia

Treatment options according to various resistant syndromes

Optimize clozapine treatment
- Check whether plasma level was ≥350 ng/mL for ≥6 months

Other additional treatment options
- Be aware that all further treatment options are poorly studied

Positive syndrome augmentation treatment
- Add on antipsychotic with additive receptor profile (eg, amisulpride, haloperidol, risperidone)
- Be aware of drug interactions

Figure 3.12 Pharmacotherapeutic algorithm for treatment-resistant schizophrenia.
These are general guidelines that must be adapted to the individual needs of each patient.
CPZ, chlorpromazine; EPS, extrapyramidal symptom; FGAs, first-generation antipsychotics;
SGAs, second-generation antipsychotics; TRS, treatment-resistant schizophrenia. Adapted from
Huber et al [11] and Lambert et al [12].

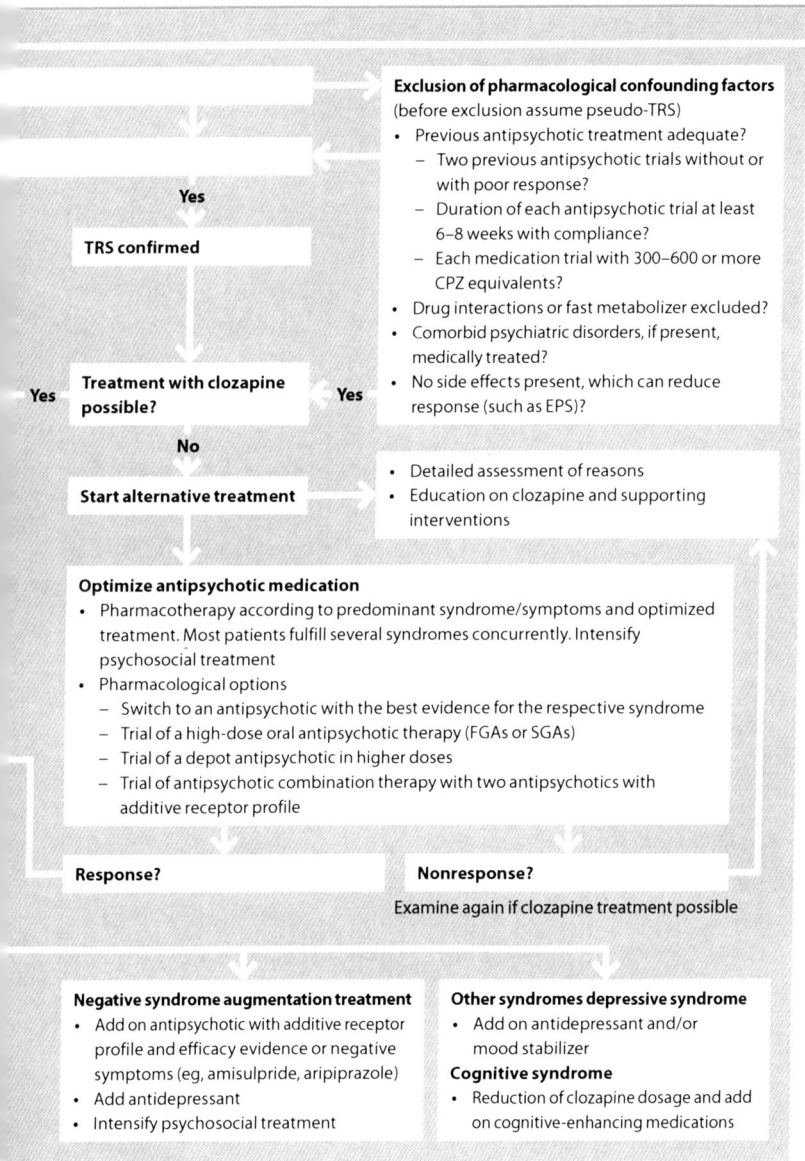

Exclusion of pharmacological confounding factors
(before exclusion assume pseudo-TRS)
- Previous antipsychotic treatment adequate?
  - Two previous antipsychotic trials without or with poor response?
  - Duration of each antipsychotic trial at least 6–8 weeks with compliance?
  - Each medication trial with 300–600 or more CPZ equivalents?
- Drug interactions or fast metabolizer excluded?
- Comorbid psychiatric disorders, if present, medically treated?
- No side effects present, which can reduce response (such as EPS)?

Yes

TRS confirmed

Yes

Treatment with clozapine possible?

Yes

No

Start alternative treatment

- Detailed assessment of reasons
- Education on clozapine and supporting interventions

Optimize antipsychotic medication
- Pharmacotherapy according to predominant syndrome/symptoms and optimized treatment. Most patients fulfill several syndromes concurrently. Intensify psychosocial treatment
- Pharmacological options
  - Switch to an antipsychotic with the best evidence for the respective syndrome
  - Trial of a high-dose oral antipsychotic therapy (FGAs or SGAs)
  - Trial of a depot antipsychotic in higher doses
  - Trial of antipsychotic combination therapy with two antipsychotics with additive receptor profile

Response?

Nonresponse?

Examine again if clozapine treatment possible

Negative syndrome augmentation treatment
- Add on antipsychotic with additive receptor profile and efficacy evidence or negative symptoms (eg, amisulpride, aripiprazole)
- Add antidepressant
- Intensify psychosocial treatment

Other syndromes depressive syndrome
- Add on antidepressant and/or mood stabilizer

Cognitive syndrome
- Reduction of clozapine dosage and add on cognitive-enhancing medications

of interventions. This includes the administration of antipsychotic medication at sufficient dosage and with sufficient compliance for at least 4–6 weeks or even longer, the successful treatment of possible comorbid psychiatric disorders, especially affective and substance abuse disorders, and concurrent management of medication side effects, especially those that can affect antipsychotic response (eg, EPS) or induce persistent symptoms (eg, depression or negative symptoms related to untreated EPS). In the case of medication nonadherence, intramuscular depot preparations, preferably SGAs, should be used. At this point, if the patient is still not responding to treatment, the clinician can proceed to stage 2.

Stage 2

After identification of the treatment-resistant domain or domain combination, the exclusion of important confounding factors and the optimization of biopsychosocial interventions, the next step is a switch to clozapine (see Figure 3.12). Clozapine is considered to be the most effective antipsychotic in TRS, which holds true with respect to both FGAs and SGAs. However, the benefits of the drug must be weighed against its serious adverse effects, including potential risks of neutropenia and agranulocytosis, weight gain, obesity and diabetes, epileptic seizures, and cardiomyopathy.

A clozapine dose of approximately 300–450 mg/day is considered to be sufficient for many patients with optimal plasma levels of 350–420 ng/mL. The dose must be raised slowly to minimize hypotension and sedation. Before determining that clozapine has not been more effective than previous treatments, it should be increased up to as much as 900 mg/day if the patient can tolerate it. No other antipsychotic drug should be given concomitantly, except during the titration period if indicated to control symptoms [25].

There are conflicting findings with respect to the necessary duration of treatment before response can be evaluated properly. In several studies, treatment-resistant patients showed strongest improvement within the first 8–12 weeks (50% of patients), whereas other studies report longer periods of 6–12 months [11,12]. There is consensus that clinicians should consider a minimum trial duration of 6 months [25,26], but they should be aware that as many as 40–70% of those treated with clozapine do not respond adequately even to an optimal treatment regimen [27].

The decision about when clozapine should be discontinued or combined with another antipsychotic is also difficult, mainly due to a lack of alternatives, negative experiences after patients were switched from clozapine back to another antipsychotic, and the fact that clozapine has additional potential effects of special importance (eg, reduction of aggressive behavior, reduced suicidality, and positive influence on tardive dyskinesia and comorbid substance abuse disorder).

If the patient refuses clozapine, it should be determined whether the patient's refusal is based on incompetence to consent to the medication. It may be that the patient is unable to appreciate the potential benefits, due to denial or lack of insight into the severity of the disease. Appropriate action to obtain guardianship may be indicated. If there has been a previous trial of clozapine, full details of what happened should be obtained: perhaps the side effects that led to premature termination of the trial were not contraindications to a retrial of clozapine. Once other treatments have been tried and the patient remains treatment resistant, it may be worth retrying clozapine with more cautious dosage escalation, avoidance of potential drug interactions, and aggressive management of the side effects. Seizures, sedation, and hypotension are side effects that might be dealt with more successfully on a second course.

If clozapine is definitely not an option, and monotherapy trials have been fully adequate, there are a number of antipsychotic combination strategies available. All have a very limited evidence base for usefulness. The pharmacotherapy at this stage depends on the affected TRS domains. For resistant positive symptoms, a primary dopamine D_2-receptor blocker (eg, risperidone, paliperidone, or haloperidol) could be combined with a "dirty" drug profile antipsychotic (multireceptor antipsychotics such as olanzapine or quetiapine); adjunctive therapy with a mood stabilizer could be an additional option. For resistant negative symptoms, adjunctive therapy with antidepressants is an option. Finally, the success of previous interventions should be reviewed and the most successful previous pharmacological intervention reinstated.

Stage 3

With respect to positive symptoms, 40–70% of those treated with clozapine monotherapy do not respond adequately despite optimal administration [27]. This condition has been designated clozapine-resistant schizophrenia, which affects approximately 10% of all patients with schizophrenia, with subsequent proportional increase with each relapse [11,12]. Before establishing the diagnosis of clozapine-resistant schizophrenia it is necessary to confirm that:

- the patient has been taking clozapine adequately for at least 6 months;
- clozapine blood levels are in the therapeutic range (≥350 ng/mL); and
- the clozapine plasma level was >350 ng/mL during the 6-month treatment period and that uncontrolled comorbid drug abuse has been absent.

If factors compromising clozapine response are ruled out, a next possible treatment step is clozapine augmentation (see Figure 3.12). However, the current body of evidence consists largely of data from smaller open trials and case reports, although data from a limited number of controlled studies are now available. In general, augmentation trials should be guided by existing evidence and a treatment plan incorporating a clear understanding of target symptoms. A means of evaluating outcome effectively needs to be in place, and the trial should be circumscribed to prevent needless polypharmacy. As a first principle, an end point needs to be established and the trial discontinued unless results confirm added benefits.

There are various augmentation strategies (see Figure 3.12), including numerous medications and electroconvulsive therapy. With respect to antipsychotics, risperidone, amisulpride, olanzapine, quetiapine, and aripiprazole have been found to have positive effects. Aripiprazole and amisulpride could also be effective, especially in the case of resistant negative symptoms. Mood stabilizers, including lithium, valproate, and lamotrigine, may be helpful in some patients. The most robust evidence for improving positive symptoms in partial responders to clozapine suggests that a course of electroconvulsive therapy is most effective.

Stage 4

Maintenance treatment with clozapine requires some specific clinical procedures:

- patients must be monitored with respect to the occurrence of agranulocytosis;
- other side effects should be monitored closely; and
- dose reduction or discontinuation of clozapine should be carried out with caution.

Agranulocytosis presents with symptoms such as fever, stomatitis, and neutropenia, with normal erythrocyte and thrombocyte count in peripheral blood. There is a higher risk of agranulocytosis for patients with previous bone marrow disorder or comedication with risk of bone marrow injury. White women aged 40 years or older who have been treated with high dosages of antipsychotics are also at high risk [28]. Of all agranulocytosis cases, 85% occurred within the first 18 weeks of treatment [29]. Therefore, current treatment requirements include weekly leukocyte counts for the first 18 weeks and once every 4 weeks subsequently. If the leukocyte count decreases or influenza-like symptoms, such as fever, sore throat, cold shivers or mouth sores, appear, an immediate total leukocyte and differential count should be carried out on an emergency basis. If it shows a leukopenia with a leukocyte count $<3500/mm^3$ or a neutrophil granulocyte count $<1500/mm^3$, clozapine must be discontinued [25]. The hematological picture generally normalizes within 2–4 weeks after discontinuation. Prognosis in agranulocytosis is better when it is detected and treated early on with hematopoietic growth factor; and the mortality is significantly lower now than it was in the past.

Clozapine has some potential side effects such as weight gain, obesity, metabolic syndrome, type 2 diabetes, epileptic seizures, and cardiomyopathy. Education about weight, diet, and exercise is recommended from the start of treatment with clozapine. Reducing or reversing the weight gain requires attention to diet and exercise as the first line of treatment. Dosage reduction may be needed to control the weight gain associated with clozapine in some but not all patients.

There have been no systematic studies of clozapine dose reduction after establishment of the optimal dose, and if dosage reduction is attempted, it should be done very gradually. Withdrawal psychosis could occur if the dose reduction is abrupt. This may be severe and unresponsive to medications other than clozapine. Therefore, whenever possible, clozapine should be tapered as another antipsychotic drug is introduced. One month of overlap is likely to minimize the risk of withdrawal psychosis.

If clozapine is stopped for more than 48 hours, it must be restarted with a dose of 12.5–25 mg and then, if there are no respiratory or cardiovascular symptoms, the dose may be quickly raised back to its previous level. If necessary, the initial dose may be higher in order to obtain relief of very severe withdrawal psychosis.

Treatment in the maintenance phase including relapse prevention

Although patients typically recover from FEP, the long-term course for many patients is still characterized by chronic illness, disability, and relapse. However, a moderately large subgroup of patients experience periods of recovery, including both adequate psychosocial functioning and the absence of major symptoms, lasting several years or longer.

The long-term, or maintenance, phase should be separated into a stabilization phase and a relapse prevention ("stable") phase. This differentiation is helpful in understanding the greater vulnerability of patients in the stabilization phase after the acute phase and the fact that many patients need a considerable period of time for complete recovery. The following points with respect to the maintenance phase, including relapse prevention, are important: the two phases are the "stabilization" phase (approximately 3–6 months after the acute phase) and the "stable" phase. The stable phase is usually associated with maintenance treatment for patients who meet criteria for being stable as well as those who continue to have persistent symptoms. General recommendations for treatment in the maintenance phase are listed in Figure 3.13.

Relapse is common in schizophrenia. During the first 5 years after initial treatment, more than 80% of patients relapse, most of them more than once [1]. Risk factors for relapse mainly include medication nonadherence and service disengagement (see Chapter 2, page 27), persistent

Recommendations for maintenance treatment of schizophrenia

General principles

- Assertive community treatment (ACT) can support service engagement and medication adherence. It could further reduce the risk of full relapse by early relapse detection and intervention. Compared with intensive case management, ACT is better in preventing relapse
- Maintenance treatment should include interventions to prevent relapse and to promote recovery, most importantly psychoeducation, family interventions, compliance therapy, cognitive–motivational addiction therapy, cognitive–behavioral therapy interventions, social skills training, and social support
- Maintenance treatment should be organized within one specialized center and provided by two clinicians (ie, case manager and physician) supported by an ACT team
- Maintenance care should further focus on
  - regular assessment of mental state including information given by relevant others
  - regular review of pharmacotherapy, including efficacy, tolerability, early detection and treatment of somatic illnesses, and risk of nonadherence
  - regular social support if needed
  - regular assessment of suicidal behavior, risk of suicide attempt and completed suicide
  - regular assessment (and treatment) of comorbid psychiatric disorders

Use of antipsychotics

- Maintenance dose range is 300–600 chlorpromazine equivalents (oral or depot) per day (<300 mg chlorpromazine equivalents/day increases risk of relapse)
- Reassessment of dosage level or need for maintenance antipsychotic therapy should be ongoing
- Continuous dosage regimens should be used: targeted, intermittent dosage maintenance strategies should not be used routinely instead of continuous dosage regimens because of increased risk of symptom worsening or relapse. Exceptions are patients who refuse maintenance or for whom some other contraindication to maintenance therapy exists, such as side-effect sensitivity
- Depot antipsychotics should be strongly considered for patients who have difficulty complying with oral medication or prefer the depot regimen; depot therapy may be used as a first-option maintenance strategy
- Duration of pharmacotherapy depends on several factors

Figure 3.13 Recommendations for maintenance treatment of schizophrenia. Adapted from Lambert et al [15].

substance use (see Chapter 2, page 38), incomplete remission within the first treatment (see page 101), cognitive deficits with reduced stress tolerance and reduced medication adherence (see Chapter 2, page 19), and inappropriate psychosocial treatment (see page 144).

Maintenance treatment with antipsychotics

The efficacy of antipsychotics in preventing relapse is uncontested, and a number of studies support this finding:

- A study of 3500 patients found that relapse rates of patients treated with placebo were 75% compared with 15% in patients treated continuously with antipsychotics [30].

- On a monthly basis, the relapse rate with placebo was 10%, compared with 2–3% seen with antipsychotic treatment [30].
- The difference in relapse rates between placebo- and antipsychotic-treated patients is approximately 50–60%, with most studies focusing on a time period of 1 to 2 years [30].
- Studies have also shown good relapse prevention in the long term: in one study patients who had remained relapse-free for 2 to 3 years had then discontinued antipsychotic treatment. Thereafter, the 1-year relapse rate was 65%, with most relapses occurring at 3–7 months after discontinuation [31,32].
- A similar relapse rate was observed in patients who had been relapse-free for 3–5 years before discontinuing antipsychotic treatment (62% relapse rate after discontinuation) [30].

Thus, accumulated evidence suggests that the vast majority of patients with schizophrenia will experience a relapse after discontinuation of antipsychotics, even after more than 5 years of successful maintenance treatment. Recommendations for the use of antipsychotics in the maintenance phase are listed in Figure 3.13.

Maintenance therapy strategies

There are three different long-term maintenance therapy strategies:

1. Continuous antipsychotic treatment with oral or depot antipsychotics in usual dosage.
2. Continuous antipsychotic treatment with oral or depot antipsychotics in low dosage.
3. The targeted or intermittent treatment strategy.

With respect to strategies 1 and 2, the decision about the optimal drug dosage during the maintenance phase can be particularly difficult, especially because the drug cannot be titrated against clinical response in the stable phase. If the dosage is too low, this may not be apparent until the patient relapses. In addition, the low-dosage strategy has not been studied with SGAs. Thus, the antipsychotic dosage in the maintenance phase should be "minimally effective," comparable to the recommendation within the acute phase.

In the third strategy, patients who are stable have their antipsychotics gradually decreased until all medication is completely discontinued. Antipsychotics are reinstituted at the earliest signs of symptomatic recurrence. Accumulated evidence suggests that intermittent treatment results in relapse rates that are twice as high as those with continuous treatment. This difference is caused mainly by difficulty in detecting early warning signs, difficulty of predicting relapse through early warning signs, and the abruptness and speed of relapse in some patients. Exceptions are patients who refuse maintenance or for whom there is some other contraindication to maintenance therapy, such as side-effect sensitivity.

Depot antipsychotics in the maintenance phase

Antipsychotics can be administered in long-acting injectable forms. There are several injectable FGAs, but only two SGAs, risperidone and olanzapine, are available in depot formulation (Figure 3.14). For a comparison of depot and oral formulations, as well as depot formulations of FGAs and SGAs, see Figure 3.3.

Duration of prevention of antipsychotic relapse

Several factors must be taken into account when considering how long the patient should be treated with medication. In general, there is a growing body of evidence suggesting the value of continuing medication for a sustained and possibly indefinite period. There are several findings that support this:

- It is still not known for how long the patient must remain stable before discontinuation of antipsychotics is safe with respect to relapse. Relapse rates after discontinuation are high in the first 2–5 years (70–90%) [33]. Following discontinuation after a 5-year stable phase the relapse rate is still above 60% [30].
- Each relapse can have several consequences for the long-term outcome and prognosis:
  - decreased response to antipsychotics with the need for higher antipsychotic dosages and the risk of increased side effects;

- a prolonged duration to reach symptomatic remission; and
- increased risk of residual symptoms with each subsequent relapse.

Taking these findings into account, general guidelines applicable to all patients are not available and would possibly be contradictory. As noted

Recommended doses of depot first- and second-generation antipsychotics in the long-term treatment of schizophrenia

Antipsychotic	Strength supplied	Dose multiplication factor*
Second-generation antipsychotics		
Risperidone microspheres	25, 37.5 and 50 mg	NA
Olanzapine pamoate	150, 210, 300 mg every 2 weeks 405 mg every 4 weeks	NA
Paliperidone palmitate	25, 50, 75, 100, 150 mg	150 mg every 4 weeks (12 mg oral paliperidone); 75 mg every 4 weeks (6 mg oral paliperidone)
First-generation antipsychotics		
Flupenthixol decanoate	20 mg/mL (2%) 100 mg/mL (10%)	3–5
Fluphenazine decanoate	25 mg/mL 100 mg/mL	2.5–6
Perphenazine enanthane	100 mg/mL	3–4
Pipotiazine palmitate	25 mg/mL 50 mg/mL	5–10
Haloperidol decanoate	50 mg/mL 100 mg/mL	15–20
Zuclopenthixol acetate	50 mg/mL 100 mg/mL	1–2
Zuclopenthixol decanoate	200 mg/mL	5–10

Figure 3.14 Recommended doses of depot first- and second-generation antipsychotics in the long-term treatment of schizophrenia. *Dosage of depot antipsychotic in relation to oral dosage (ie, previous oral dosage x multiplication factor). Adapted from Lambert et al [15].

earlier, the decision about how long a patient should take an antipsychotic should be made together with the patient and relatives, taking into account not only current knowledge about relapse prevention but also the personal context of the patient (eg, psychiatric history, comorbidity, and knowledge about early warning signs).

Dosage interval	Dosage in the long-term treatment (mg/pro DI)	Highest possible dosage (mg/pro DI)
• Every 2 weeks • Onset of action after 3 weeks • Peak plasma level: 4–6 weeks	• 25–50	50
• Every 2–4 weeks	• 150–405 every 2–4 weeks	300 every 2 weeks
• Every 4 weeks (150 mg as first deltoid application, 100 mg after 8 days of deltoid application; then 25–150 mg deltoid or gluteal application)	• 25–150 every 4 weeks; recommended dose: 75 every 4 weeks	150 every 4 weeks
• Every 2–3 weeks • Initial recommended dose: 20 mg • Peak plasma level: 4–7 days	• 20–60	100
• Every 4 weeks • Initial dose: 2.5–12.5 mg • First peak plasma level: 8–12 hours • Second peak plasma level: 8–12 days	• 6.25–25 every 2–3 weeks • 25–50 every 4 weeks	100
• Every 2–3 weeks • Peak plasma level: 2–3 days	• 50–200	200
• Every 4 weeks • Peak plasma level: 12–24 hours	• 50–250	300
• Every 4 weeks • Peak plasma level: 3–9 days	• Symptom suppression: 100–200 • Prophylaxis: 25–150	300
• Every 1–3 days • Peak plasma level: 36 hours	• 50–150	200
• Every 2–4 weeks • Peak plasma level: 4–7 days	• 100–350	400

From a risk–benefit perspective, actual and possible future side effects should also be taken into account. Several expert consensus guidelines recommend that patients with first-episode psychosis should be maintained on an antipsychotic for 12–24 months after remission of psychotic symptoms. This recommendation is also applicable for children and adolescents with schizophrenia. Nevertheless, studies suggest that there is a relapse risk of 70–90% within the first 5 years of FEP, and that those patients who discontinue antipsychotic medication have the highest risk. In reverse, it can be argued that approximately 20% of the patients would remain well without maintenance antipsychotic treatment. However, identifying patients who do not need ongoing antipsychotic treatment in the long term is difficult. Although some patient and illness characteristics appear to indicate a lower risk of future relapse, criteria of definitive prognostic relevance are still lacking; no predictor alone or in combination with others allows a dependable prognosis. As a general rule, patients with two or more relapses may be treated with standard dosages for prolonged periods of up to 5 years or longer.

Discontinuing antipsychotic treatment

Patients discontinuing antipsychotics abruptly have a 50% higher risk of relapse within the next 6 months than patients who discontinue medication by slow reduction over 6–9 months. The dosage should not be decreased by more than 20% within a period of 4–8 weeks [34]. During this phase of reduction and discontinuation, psychotherapeutic measures should be intensified. After discontinuation, all patients need ongoing treatment, including close monitoring and easy access to services, in case a relapse appears possible.

Management of significant side effects and physical illness

Martin Lambert

General considerations

Compared with the general population, people with schizophrenia have a lifespan that is up to 20% shorter; for example in the USA it is approximately 15–20 years shorter. This is associated mainly with a higher prevalence of life-shortening physical diseases such as CVD, smoking, obesity, dyslipidemia, hypertension, metabolic syndrome, type 2 diabetes, HIV infections, and hepatitis, and by health services often failing to prevent, detect, and treat these physical diseases at both early and later stages. The increased frequency of physical diseases in schizophrenia might be the result of factors related to the illness itself (eg, smoking, reduced physical activity, poor nutrition, drug or alcohol use, functioning level, symptoms and stigma, which aggravate access to care) and its treatment (eg, antipsychotic or polypharmacological treatment with possible side effects such as weight gain, obesity, or metabolic syndrome). There are several possible approaches to dealing with this problem:

- awareness and education programs on physical diseases in schizophrenia for students, psychiatrists, primary care physicians, patients, and relatives;
- implementation of an integrated network of psychiatrists and primary care physicians;
- improved access to medical care for people with schizophrenia; and
- consequent clinical implementation of already existing treatment guidelines.

Optimal management of side effects is one requirement for the prevention of life-shortening physical illnesses. Here, the clinician has to separate tolerability and safety issues. Tolerability issues can be defined in relation to nonlethal, time-limited or manageable adverse events (eg, mild parkinsonism, nausea, or sedation), whereas safety issues can be defined as life-threatening, treatment-related adverse events that can occur on an acute or chronic basis (eg, NMS or metabolic syndrome). Some side effects can start as a tolerability issue (eg, weight gain) and could become a safety issue later on (weight gain can lead to obesity, which can lead to metabolic syndrome and diabetes).

All antipsychotics have the potential to produce adverse effects of different prevalence and severity. Each adverse event can be subjectively distressing and therefore has the potential to diminish patients' wellbeing (for side effects of all SGAs and some FGAs see Figure 3.15).

Selected side effects of commonly used antipsychotics

Type of side effect*	Haloperidol	Amisulpride	Aripiprazole	Clozapine	Olanzapine	Quetiapine IR/XR	Paliperidone	Risperidone	Ziprasidone
Akathisia/parkinsonism	+++	0–+	+	0	0–+	0–+	0–++	0–++	0–+
Tardive dyskinesia	+++	(+)	?	0	(+)	?	(+)	(+)	?
Seizures	+	0	(+)	++	0	0	0	0	0
QT prolongation	+	(+)	0 (?)	(+)	(+)	(+)	(+)	(+)	+
Glucose abnormalities	(+)	(+)	0	+++	+++	++	++	++	0
Dyslipidemia	(+)	(+)	0	+++	+++	++	++	++	0
Constipation	+	++	0	+++	++	+	++	++	0
Hypotension	++	0	+	+	(+)	++	++	++	+
Agranulocytosis	0	0	0	+	0	0	0	0	0
Weight gain†	+	+	+	+++	+++	++	++	++	0–+
Prolactin elevation	+++	+++	0	0	(+)	(+)	++	++	(+)
Galactorrhea	++	++	0	0	0	0	++	++	0
Dys-/amenorrhea	++	++	0	0	0	(+)	++	++	0
Sedation	+++	0–+	0	+++	+++	++	+	+	0–(+)
Malignant neuroleptic syndrome	(+)	?	(+)	(+)	(+)	(+)	(+)	(+)	?

Figure 3.15 Selected side effects of commonly used antipsychotics. Frequency and severity of side effects refers to information obtained by pharmaceutical companies, FDA, additional literature, and various guidelines (eg, American Psychiatric Association, Canadian Psychiatric Association). *0, no risk; (+), occasionally, may be no difference to placebo; +, mild (<1%); ++, sometimes (<10%); +++, frequently (>10%); ?, not stated possibly due to lack of data. †Weight gain during 6–10 weeks: +, low (0–1.5 kg); ++, medium (1.5–3 kg); +++, high (>3 kg). ER, extended release; FDA, US Food and Drug Administration; IR, immediate release. Adapted from Lambert et al [15].

Extrapyramidal motor side effects

Acute EPS (parkinsonism, akathisia, acute dyskinesia, and dystonia) should be considered separately from those side effects that occur only after months or years of antipsychotic treatment (eg, tardive dyskinesia; Figure 3.16). Current knowledge about EPS can be summarized as follows:

- 50–70% of patients taking FGAs experience a clinically significant degree of acute EPS [3,35], which are sometimes only subjectively detectable but are often combined with great distress. Antipsychotic-induced parkinsonism affects 10–80% of patients taking FGAs, and akathisia affects up to 30% [2].

- Antipsychotic-naïve patients have a higher sensitivity to EPS, with a prevalence of 70–80% [36].

- SGAs generally have a lower propensity to induce EPS. With some SGAs the prevalence of EPS is comparable to placebo across the complete dose range; in others the risk of EPS is dose-dependent.

- Compared with haloperidol, all SGAs require less concomitant administration of anticholinergic drugs.

- Acute EPS can have several consequences:
  - reduced response to antipsychotic medication;
  - impaired subjective wellbeing and quality of life;
  - cognitive dysfunctions, associated either directly through motor disturbances or indirectly through additional anticholinergic drugs;
  - higher risk of developing tardive dyskinesia;
  - higher risk of medication nonadherence;

Acute extrapyramidal motor side effects

Side effects	Acute dyskinesia or dystonia	Parkinsonism	Akathisia
Prevalence*	• Dyskinesia: 5% • Dystonia: up to 25% • Depending on type and dose of antipsychotic • 50% in first 2 days, 90% in first 4–5 days	• 15–35% • 50–75% within first 4 weeks • 90% within first 3 month	• 20–25% • 50% within first 4 weeks • 90% within first 2 or 3 months
Cause	Increased dopamine synthesis[†]	Dopaminergic hypoactivity or cholinergic hyperactivity	Blockade of mesocortical dopaminergic receptors[†]

Figure 3.16 Acute extrapyramidal motor side effects (continues overleaf).

Side effects	Acute dyskinesia or dystonia	Parkinsonism	Akathisia
Risk factors	• Children/adolescents • Antipsychotic naïve • High-potency antipsychotic • High initial dosage • Rapid dosage increase • Reduction of initially high dosage • Re-exposure to antipsychotic that previously induced EPS • Previous EPS	• Children/adolescents • Antipsychotic naïve • Female/male = 2:1 • Elderly patients • High-potency antipsychotic • High initial dosage • Rapid dosage increase • Reduction of initially high dosage • Re-exposure to antipsychotic that previously induced EPS • Previous EPS	• Children/adolescents • Antipsychotic naïve • High-potency antipsychotic • High initial dosage • Rapid dosage increase • Re-exposure to antipsychotic that previously induced EPS • Previous EPS
Clinical presentation	• Abnormal movements of head and neck (eg, retrocollis or torticollis) • Cramped masseter muscles (locked jaw, mouth pulled open, grimacing, trismus) • Difficulties swallowing (dysphagia), speaking, or breathing (cramped hyopharyngeal muscle, dysphonia) • Slurred or unclear speech, due to dysarthria and macroglossia • Extended or dysfunctional tongue • Ocular cramp or cramped closure of eyelid (oculogyric crisis) • Opisthotonos	• Hypokinesia/akinesia: lack of movement, animia (mask face), monotone voice, hypersalivation, reduced associated movement of arms • Rigidity: increased muscle tone, usually symmetrical, affecting arms and legs; cogwheel phenomenon • Tremor: slow rhythm tremor, with frequency of 3–6 beats/s, affecting extremities, head, mouth and tongue; rabbit syndrome • Cognitive and emotional impairments	• Subjective: feeling of unrest, inability to relax, anxiety, nervousness, irritation • Objective: unable to sit still, festinating gait, stamping, recurring movements of arms and legs, pacing to alleviate unrest

Figure 3.16 Acute extrapyramidal motor side effects (continues opposite).

Side effects	Acute dyskinesia or dystonia	Parkinsonism	Akathisia
Clinical consequences	• Perceived as agonizing • Influences future compliance • Speech difficulties • Swallowing difficulties • Risk of suffocation	• Reduced capability to move and think impairs rehabilitation • Stigmatization • Differential evaluation to negative or depressive symptoms not easy • Associated with poor response	• Perceived as agonizing • Influences future compliance • Differential evaluation to psychotic agitation not easy
Prevention and treatment	• Use of second-generation antipsychotics • Initial treatment with low dosage • Slow dosage increase • No rapid reduction • Lowest effective dosage • Intravenous application of benzatropine (inject slowly, symptoms disappear within 10–30 min) • Oral treatment: adults 1–3 sustained-release tablets daily; children (3–15 years) 1–2 mg benzatropine one to three times daily • Antipsychotic dose adjustment • Switch of antipsychotic	• Use of second-generation antipsychotics • Initial treatment with low dosage • Slow dosage increase • No rapid reduction • Lowest effective dosage • Use of anticholinergics	• Use of second-generation antipsychotics • Initial treatment with low dosage • Slow dosage increase • No rapid reduction • Lowest effective dosage • Use of propranolol 30–80 mg/day • Use of benzodiazepines

Figure 3.16 Acute extrapyramidal motor side effects (continued). EPS, extrapyramidal symptoms. *With respect to all patients receiving antipsychotic treatment. [†]Not yet securely established. Adapted from Lambert et al [15].

- social consequences, especially stigmatization; and
- high risk of misdiagnosis (eg, parkinsonism as depression, akathisia as psychotic agitation).

Parkinsonism is an EPS that is most commonly treated with the administration of anticholinergic drugs (eg, biperiden or benzatropine). Beta-blockers, such as propranolol, and benzodiazepines are used to treat akathisia.

Tardive dyskinesia

Tardive dyskinesia is a neurologic syndrome caused by the use of antipsychotic drugs. Repetitive, involuntary, purposeless movements such as grimacing, tongue protrusion, lip smacking, puckering and pursing, and rapid eye blinking characterizes tardive dyskinesia. Movements of the arms, legs, and trunk may also occur. Involuntary movements of the fingers may appear as if the patient is playing an invisible guitar or piano. Diagnosis of antipsychotic-induced tardive dyskinesia requires a patient to meet certain criteria, and exclusion of other possible syndromes through differential diagnosis (Figure 3.17). There are populations that are especially at risk for tardive dyskinesia, listed in Figure 3.18.

Tardive dyskinesia: diagnostic criteria and differential diagnosis

Diagnostic criteria according to Schooler and Kane

- At least 3 months of cumulative antipsychotic exposure
- At least moderate abnormal involuntary movements in one or more body area or mild movements in two or more body areas
- The absence of differential diagnoses that produce involuntary hyperkinetic dyskinesias

Most important differential diagnosis

- Withdrawal TD after discontinuation of antipsychotics (in many cases TD already existed and was suppressed by antipsychotic treatment)
- Other movement disorders (eg, Parkinson's disease, Pisa or rabbit syndrome, Gilles de la Tourette's syndrome)
- Spontaneous hyperkinesias, often among older women
- Hyperkinesias related to other disorders (eg, Wilson's disease or Huntington's disease)
- Hyperkinesias related to other medications (eg, L-dopa, tricyclic antidepressants, lithium, antihistamines, anticonvulsants, phenytoin, metoclopramide, buspirone, flunarizine, selective serotonin reuptake inhibitors, anticholinergic drugs)
- Other differential diagnoses (eg, grimaces, stereotypes and mannerisms as part of schizophrenic psychosis, psychomotor symptoms for agitated depression)

Figure 3.17 Tardive dyskinesia: diagnostic criteria and differential diagnosis. TD, tardive dyskinesia. Adapted from Schooler et al [37].

Populations at risk of tardive dyskinesia

Population	Potential reason
Older patients	Rate of TD increases with age (50% in a group of elderly schizophrenic patients)
Elderly women	Decreased estrogen levels and increased phenylalanine levels
Patients who have used DRAs for >3 months	Increased exposure to DRAs
Patients with diabetes, independent of use of DRAs (risk increases with DRA use)	Impaired glucose metabolism
Patients with previous drug-induced parkinsonism	Not related to the use of anticholinergic drugs
People with phenylketonuria	Increased phenylalanine levels

Figure 3.18 Populations at risk of tardive dyskinesia. DRAs, dopamine-receptor antagonists; TD, tardive dyskinesia.

Current evidence supports a lower tardive dyskinesia risk with SGAs than with FGAs (annual incidence of 3.9% for SGAs and 5.5% for FGAs) [38]. The rate of tardive dyskinesia increases with age, as does the rate of spontaneous dyskinesias. Risk for tardive dyskinesia is 0.35% in children taking SGAs; 2.98% in adults taking SGAs compared with 7.7% in those taking FGAs; and 5.2% in elderly patients taking SGAs compared with 5.2% in those taking FGAs. In a middle-aged population of 40- to 45-year-old patients with schizophrenia, the prevalence of tardive dyskinesia was 13.1%, 15.6%, and 32.4% for patients treated with SGAs, antipsychotic-free patients, and those treated with FGAs, respectively [38].

There is no standard treatment for tardive dyskinesia. Usually, the treatment is difficult, lengthy, and generally based on disease severity (Figure 3.19). In many cases the causative medication is adjusted to the lowest possible dose, or discontinued if at all possible. However, for many patients with a severe underlying condition this may not be a feasible option. Replacing the antipsychotic drug with other medications (eg, SGAs) may help some patients, especially those who were treated with FGAs. Treatment with clozapine is another promising option. Other drugs such as vitamin E or B_6, benzodiazepines, adrenergic antagonists, and dopamine agonists may also be beneficial (Figure 3.19).

Symptoms of tardive dyskinesia may remain even after the medication is stopped. Data on the long-term course of tardive dyskinesia suggest that approximately 40% of patients show a worsening of symptoms over time. The remaining 50–60% show less severe symptoms with no progression or remission [39]. However, with careful management, some symptoms may improve or disappear with time. Prevention of tardive dyskinesia includes early recognition and the prescription of SGAs in the lowest possible dose. In all cases, for antipsychotic medication to be prescribed, the benefits of taking it should be judged to outweigh the risks of developing tardive dyskinesia.

Recommendations for treatment of tardive dyskinesia

Mild-to-moderate tardive dyskinesia, no symptom suppression required

- Re-evaluate the necessity for antipsychotic treatment (relapse/TD ratio). Be aware that complete and permanent reversibility of TD is rare. The clinical feasibility of antipsychotic withdrawal is severely limited by the high risk of psychotic relapse
- Adjust dose to the lowest possible if antipsychotic has to be maintained; otherwise consider switching to SGAs (eg, quetiapine or olanzapine)*
- If symptoms persist after switching to SGAs, consider concurrent treatment with tiapride over 6–12 weeks (600 mg/day)
- If symptoms persist, consider symptom suppression treatment with SGAs (see below)
- If symptoms persist, consider switch to clozapine and follow guidelines for severe TD

Severe tardive dyskinesia, symptom suppression required

- Adjust dose to the lowest possible if antipsychotic has to be maintained. Be aware that severe TD is often concurrent with severe (chronic) courses of schizophrenia and that risk of relapse with dose reduction is high
- Consider switching to SGAs (eg, quetiapine or olanzapine), increasing the dose gradually until symptoms of TD are suppressed
- If symptoms persist after TD suppression with SGAs, consider concurrent treatment with tiapride over 6–12 weeks (600 mg/day)
- If symptoms persist, switch to clozapine. Wait 6–12 months before symptoms of TD are judged to be chronic
- The following drugs could be added to SGAs or clozapine. Their effects are relatively uncertain and some of these drugs only protect against deterioration of TD rather than improve symptoms of TD:
  - vitamin E (1200–1600 IU/day) over a period of 3 months[†]
  - vitamin B_6 (400 mg/day)
  - calcium channel blocker (eg, nifedipine 40–80 mg/day)
  - α_2-agonist (eg, clonidine)
  - benzodiazepine
  - amine-depleting drugs (eg, reserpine, tetrabenazine): block reuptake of dopamine, norepinephrine, and serotonin, thereby depleting central availability of these neurotransmitters. Significant side effects limit the use of these drugs

Figure 3.19 Recommendations for treatment of tardive dyskinesia. *Worsening of TD can occur if high-potency FGAs are switched to SGAs. [†] Newer reviews indicate that vitamin E protects against deterioration of TD, but there is no evidence that vitamin E improves symptoms of TD. FGAs, first-generation antipsychotics; SGAs, second-generation antipsychotics; TD, tardive dyskinesia. Adapted from Lambert et al [15].

Neuroleptic malignant syndrome

The rare occurrence of NMS (sometimes known as malignant neuroleptic syndrome) is characterized by hyperthermia and severe muscle rigidity after intake of antipsychotics. These primary symptoms are accompanied by at least five of the following symptoms (relevant for diagnosis; Figure 3.20): severe hyperhidrosis, dysphagia, tremor, incontinence, reduced consciousness (from confusion to stupor up to coma),

Symptoms and diagnostic criteria of neuroleptic malignant syndrome	
Syndrome	**Possible symptoms**
Extrapyramidal motor side effects	• Hypokinesia/akinesia, muscle rigidity (typically evident) • Tremor • Hyporeflexia • Opisthotonos, trismus • Oculogyric crisis
Vegetative symptoms	• Hyperthermia (>38°C) • Tachycardia, increased blood pressure • Incontinence
Psychic symptoms	• Stupor • Confusion • Mutism • Impaired consciousness • Catatonia
Conspicuous lab findings	• Creatine kinase and liver enzyme elevation • Myoglobinuria (in case of rhabdomyolysis) • Leukocytosis • Metabolic acidosis
Diagnostic criteria	

- Antipsychotic treatment in the last 4 weeks
- Hyperthermia (>38°C)
- Muscle rigidity
- Existence of at least five of the following symptoms:
  - severe hyperhidrosis
  - dysphagia
  - tremor
  - incontinence
  - reduced consciousness
  - mutism
  - tachycardia
  - increased or fluctuating blood pressure
  - leukocytosis
  - laboratory findings indicating muscle injury
- Exclusion of other reasons

Figure 3.20 Symptoms and diagnostic criteria of neuroleptic malignant syndrome. Adapted from Lambert et al [15].

mutism, tachycardia, increased or fluctuating blood pressure, leukocytosis (10,000–20,000 white blood cells/µL; present in 50% of patients), and laboratory findings indicating muscle injury (such as increased creatine phosphokinase >300 U/L, present in only 50% of the cases) [40,41]. Muscle cramps, fasciculation, or opisthotonos are also observed occasionally. Pathological laboratory findings are defined as an increased blood sedimentation rate as well as an increase in aspartate transaminase and alanine transaminase due to the increased rigidity.

Furthermore, a tachypnea with metabolic acidosis can occur, sometimes with respiratory insufficiency. Urine of patients with NMS can be dark due to myoglobinuria. The syndrome can be accompanied by agitation or acute dystonic reactions. For the diagnosis it is important to ascertain that symptoms are not due to the consumption of other medications (eg, phencyclidine), neurologic or other disorders (eg, viral encephalitis), or even another psychiatric disorder such as disorders with catatonic symptoms, especially schizophrenia.

Studies on the frequency of NMS report a prevalence of 0.02–2.4% [42,43]. It occurs mostly under treatment with high-potency FGAs; however, SGAs (eg, clozapine, risperidone, olanzapine, zotepine, or quetiapine) have also been reported to cause NMS. It usually develops in the early phase of antipsychotic treatment. Most cases develop within the first 4 weeks, with two-thirds appearing in the first week, yet cases may develop even after months of treatment. NMS most often develops in young male patients. Other risk factors include previous NMS, rapid dosage increase, concurrent dehydration, parenteral antipsychotic treatment, an anxious–depressive agitation, previous cerebral injuries, and combination treatment with medications, which can induce NMS (eg, lithium, carbamazepine, tricyclic antidepressants, selective serotonin reuptake inhibitors, or selective norepinephrine reuptake inhibitors).

Differential diagnoses include the serotonin syndrome, malignant hyperthermia, allergic medication reactions, heatstroke, hypokinetic crisis in Parkinson's disease, infections of the central nervous system, toxic encephalopathia, and febrile catatonia.

The most important causal intervention is to stop the antipsychotic treatment immediately. All other interventions focus on the somatic symptoms of NMS and aim to reduce life-threatening complications. After discontinuation of antipsychotic treatment, NMS gradually goes into remission within 2 weeks for oral medication and 4 weeks for depot medication; the average duration of NMS is 5 days [40,41]. In 5–20% of cases NMS has proved fatal [40,41], which is mainly due to secondary complications such as renal failure (myoglobinemia with the risk of developing a crush syndrome), respiratory insufficiency, and cardiac and circulatory failure. Treatment in an intensive care unit is usually necessary and highly recommended.

In most cases, antipsychotic treatment has to be restarted after NMS is in remission. A previous NMS is, however, the most powerful predictor for a subsequent NMS. As such, the next antipsychotic has to be started at a low dose and should be increased slowly, comedications that can induce NMS should be avoided, and patients should be monitored closely in the first 4 weeks of treatment (eg, for signs of hyperthermia and rigidity, and creatine kinase levels).

Weight gain and obesity

People with schizophrenia are more likely to be overweight or obese than the general population. It has been estimated that obesity affects 45–55% of patients at levels that lead to body weight exceeding the ideal by 20% or more [44]. Extreme weight gain of 10–20 kg occurs in approximately 10–20% of cases [44] (see Figure 3.21 for a classification of obesity and classification of waist circumferences, and Figure 3.22 for assessment of body mass index). Besides the degree of obesity, the fat distribution pattern is also an important factor for the risk of metabolic syndrome and CVD (Figure 3.21).

Weight gain is a multifactorial occurrence related to various general factors and to factors related to the illness itself as well as its treatment (Figures 3.23 and 3.24). Many antipsychotics and other psychotropic medications can cause weight gain, although prevalence and extent of weight gain vary from drug to drug (Figure 3.25). Predictors of weight gain are poorly understood. Besides the previously described causes, the following predictors are known in schizophrenia: increased appetite directly after start of drug treatment, good clinical response, low baseline body mass index (<23), younger age, and concurrent treatment with other medications that induce weight gain. The time course of the weight gain is also poorly researched, but the highest weight gain appears to occur in the first 6–9 months of antipsychotic treatment, mainly in the first 12 weeks [46,47].

Category	BMI (kg/m^2)	Risk for metabolic and cardiovascular diseases
Underweight	<18.5	Low
Normal weight	18.5–24.9	Average
Overweight	≥25.0	
Preobesity	25–29.9	Marginally increased
Obesity degree I	30–34.9	Increased
Obesity degree II	35–39.9	High
Obesity degree III	≥40	Very high

Classification of the waist circumference with the related risk for metabolic and cardiovascular diseases	Waist circumference (cm)	
	Male	Female
Increased	≥94	≥80
Considerably increased	≥102	≥88

Figure 3.21 Classification of risk for metabolic and cardiovascular disease according to weight and waist circumference in adults. Adapted from The National Institutes of Health [45].

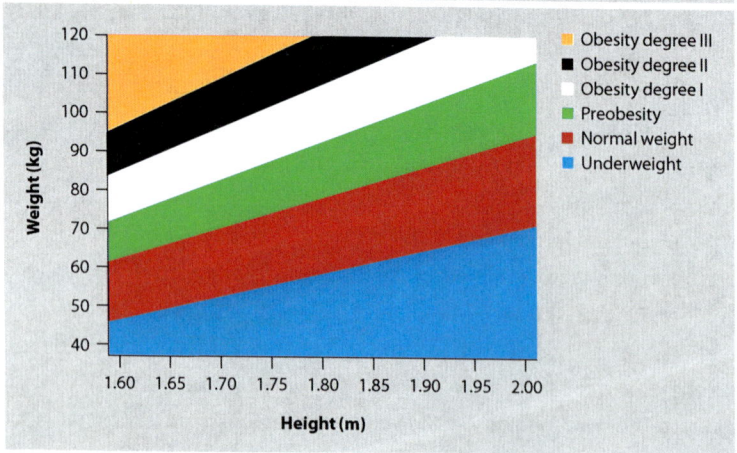

Figure 3.22 Classification of weight according of the body mass index. Adapted from Lambert [7].

Causes of weight gain in patients with schizophrenia

General causes

- Familial disposition, genetic causes
- Lifestyle (reduced exercise, poor nutrition)
- Chronic stress
- Eating disorder (eg, binge-eating disorder, bulimia)
- Endocrine disorders (eg, hypothyroidism, Cushing's syndrome)
- Medications (eg, some antidepressants, antipsychotics, and medications against hypertension)
- Other causes (eg, pregnancy, cessation of nicotine use)

Specific causes in patients with schizophrenia

- Antipsychotics that cause weight gain (for mechanism of antipsychotic-induced weight gain, see Figure 3.24)
- Combinations of medications that can cause weight gain
- Symptoms and consequences of schizophrenia, which can cause inactivity and decrease the ability to live healthily (eg, negative symptoms, depression, reduced functional level, reduced financial resources)

Figure 3.23 Causes of weight gain in patients with schizophrenia. Causes of weight gain in general and specifically for patients with schizophrenia. Adapted from Lambert [7].

Among SGAs, clozapine and olanzapine have a fairly high potential for causing weight gain, especially if combined with other psychotropic drugs that have high weight-gain potential. To a lesser extent, zotepine, risperidone, paliperidone, quetiapine, and amisulpride have some potential to cause weight gain, whereas ziprasidone and aripiprazole hardly affect body weight (Figure 3.25). Contrary to earlier beliefs, several FGAs also have a potential to induce weight gain. The risk of weight gain related to treatment with low-potency FGAs or chlorpromazine is lower compared with clozapine and olanzapine; whereas the risk with haloperidol, perphenazine, and fluphenazine, at least in the short term, is comparable to ziprasidone (ie, low). However, some long-term studies have found considerable weight gain with haloperidol and other FGAs.

Various diseases are associated with obesity: metabolic syndrome, type 2 diabetes, hypertension, dyslipidemia, and CVD (Figure 3.26). However, the consequences are not only somatic; adherence, subjective wellbeing, self-esteem, social functioning, stigmatization, and quality of life are also affected by being overweight or obese. Therefore, clinicians should alert patients and their caregivers to the health risk associated with excess weight and encourage patients to self-monitor their weight

Mechanism of antipsychotic-induced weight gain

Effects on the basic metabolic rate

- Antipsychotics, such as clozapine, can reduce basal metabolic rate and thereby energy expenditure. For other antipsychotics with increased weight gain risk, this direct association has not been found (eg, olanzapine)

Effects on receptors

- Antagonism of 5-HT$_{2C}$ and histamine H$_1$-receptors can induce increased appetite and thereby weight gain. Further, H$_1$-receptor blockade can interfere with appetite-reducing effects of leptin
- Clozapine and olanzapine show a strong affinity to both receptors and are associated with a high risk of weight gain
- Risperidone shows a lower affinity and is associated with a lower risk of weight gain
- Ziprasidone shows a high affinity for 5-HT$_{1A}$ and 5-HT$_{2C}$ receptors. Its weight-neutral profile is explained by synaptic inhibition of serotonin and norepinephrine reuptake
- Aripiprazole shows a partial D$_2$-receptor and 5-HT$_{1A}$-receptor agonism and 5-HT$_{2A}$-receptor antagonism. Its weight-neutral profile is explained by lack of 5-HT$_{2C}$-receptor antagonism
- Other less well-researched receptors may also be involved (eg, α_2-adrenergic and SREBP-1)

Pharmacogenetic findings

- Patients with low BMI show greatest weight gain. Early and fast weight gain is a well-known predictor for the degree of long-term weight gain. Both findings support pharmacogenetic influences
- 5-HT$_{2C}$-receptor promoter region polymorphism (759C/T variant) shows strong association with weight gain and increased risk for metabolic syndrome. The underlying hypothesis postulates an interaction with the circulating leptin level

Leptin

- Leptin is coded by the "obese" gene and is produced in fat cells. Its receptors are located in two different brain regions: nucleus arcuatus and nucleus paraventricularis of the hypothalamus. With reduction of fat depots in the body, the level of circulating leptin is reduced, which results in increased appetite. However, newer studies have demonstrated that obese people have increased levels of leptin, which shows that obesity can cause leptin resistance, where the effect of leptin on the brain regions is reduced
- Several studies have shown that antipsychotics can influence leptin secretion, circulating leptin level, and leptin resistance. However, they did not control for the level of obesity. Studies that controlled for obesity have found a positive correlation for the degree of obesity, gender and leptin secretion. The association between antipsychotic treatment and leptin is not fully understood yet

Ghreline

- Ghreline (growth hormone-release-inducing hormone) is an appetite-increasing hormone, produced in the gastric mucosa, which stimulates the secretion of neuropeptide Y. Neuropeptide Y itself increases food intake and possibly decreases anxiety and depression. The influence of antipsychotics on ghreline secretion is currently unclear. Some studies found no antipsychotic-increased secretion of ghreline; others, on olanzapine, found an increased secretion

Weight gain through indirect effects on glucose and lipids

- Hyperglycemia and hyperlipidemia are seen as consequences of weight gain and obesity. There are, however, studies that have found hyperglycemia and hyperlipidemia independent of the degree of obesity (eg, for olanzapine or clozapine). Through increased insulin resistance, some antipsychotics are associated with a higher risk of type 2 diabetes. Dyslipidemia itself causes insulin resistance, which leads to an increase of adipose tissue. Correspondingly, there is a complex association of antipsychotics, hyperglycemia, hyperlipidemia and weight gain

Figure 3.24 Mechanism of antipsychotic-induced weight gain. 5-HT, serotonin; BMI, body mass index; D, dopamine; H, histamine; SREBP, sterol regulatory element-binding protein. Adapted from Newcomer et al [48].

Degree of weight gain with different antipsychotics and other psychotropic medications within the first 3 months of treatment

	Weight		
	High	**Average**	**Low**
Antidepressants	Amitrlptyline Doxepine Maprotiline Mirtazapine Trimipramine	Clomipramine Imipramine Nortriptyline	Citalopram Fluoxetine Fluvoxamine Sertraline
Antipsychotics	Clozapine Olanzapine	Chlorpromazine Paliperidone Quetiapine IR or XR Risperidone Zotepine Zuclopenthixol	Amisulpride Aripiprazole Fluanxol Fluphenazine Haloperidol/ ziprasidone
Mood stabilizers	Lithium Valproate	Carbamazepine	Gabapentine Lamotrigine Topiramate

Figure 3.25 Degree of weight gain with different antipsychotics and other psychotropic medications within the first 3 months of treatment. Adapted from Lambert [7].

and other risk factors (Figure 3.27). The management of weight gain, once it has occurred, involves a multidisciplinary approach (Figure 3.27). Switching to antipsychotics with a lower potential for inducing weight gain can help. The reduction of weight is possibly greatest if an antipsychotic with no risk of weight gain is combined with a specific weight-loss intervention and physical training. Recommendations for treatment of weight gain are given in Figure 3.27.

Metabolic syndrome and cardiovascular disorders

The metabolic syndrome is defined by the presence of three or more cardiometabolic risk factors associated with insulin resistance, including abdominal obesity, dyslipidemia, elevated blood pressure, and glucose intolerance (Figure 3.28). A special aspect of the metabolic syndrome is insulin resistance, which is a state that precedes development of type 2 diabetes. Type 2 diabetes occurs after a prolonged period of metabolic syndrome if the pancreas is unable to compensate for the reduced insulin effect by increased insulin distribution. There is often a delay between the occurrence of the metabolic syndrome and the onset of type 2 diabetes, which opens the possibility of early detection. The early

Weight gain and obesity in schizophrenia: consequences and complications

- Carbohydrate metabolism dysfunctions (eg, insulin resistance, type 2 diabetes)
- Dyslipidemia
- Hyperuricemia/gout
- Hemostasis dysfunctions
- Chronic inflammation
- Hypertension, left ventricular hypertrophy
- Cardiovascular diseases (eg, coronary heart disease, stroke, cardiac insufficiency)
- Increased cancer risk (in females: endometrium, cervix, ovarian, breast, kidney, colon; in males: prostate, colon, gallbladder, pancreas, liver, kidney, esophagus)
- Hormonal dysfunctions
- Pulmonary dysfunctions (eg, dyspnea, hypoventilation, sleep apnea syndrome)
- Gastrointestinal diseases (eg, fat liver, fat liver hepatitis, reflux disease)

Degenerative diseases of the musculoskeletal system

- Increased operation and anesthesia risk
- General disturbances (eg, increased sweating, exposure dyspnea)
- Decreased activity
- Reduced quality of life
- Increased accident hazard
- Increased complication during pregnancy and birth
- Psychosocial consequences such as depression, anxiety, stigmatization, self-worth problems, social isolation
- Reduced medication compliance

Figure 3.26 Weight gain and obesity in schizophrenia: consequences and complications.
Adapted from Lambert [7].

diagnosis of disturbed glucose tolerance is possible only through an oral glucose tolerance test. Testing fasting glucose or glycated hemoglobin is indicated only to monitor already existing type 2 diabetes.

Patients with schizophrenia in general, and especially those on continuous antipsychotic medication, have a higher risk of metabolic syndrome [50]:

- 17% in first episode (duration of illness <1.5 years);
- 28.5% in short-term illness (1.5–10 years);
- 42.4% in subchronically ill patients (10–20 years); and
- 49.4% in chronically ill patients (>20 years).

In the age range of 35–45 years the risk of metabolic syndrome in schizophrenia is threefold higher than in the general population, and in the range of 45–55 years it is twofold higher [50]. As shown in the Clinical Antipsychotic Trials of Intervention Effectiveness (CATIE) study, females have a higher risk compared with males (51.6% vs 36.0%, respectively) [51]. Patients with the following risk factors have the highest risk for metabolic syndrome: older age, women during menopause, lower income, poor nutrition, and physical inactivity (Figure 3.29).

Weight gain and obesity in schizophrenia: prevention and treatment

Recommendations for prevention

The need for prevention is related to the following clinical findings:
- With increased duration and severity of obesity, treatment gets more complex and is associated with a lower chance of weight reduction
- The somatic and psychosocial after, effects of obesity are mostly irreversible
- The prevalence of obesity in most industrial nations is so high that the economic health resources are no longer sufficient
- The psychosocial consequences of schizophrenia may reduce the ability to participate in weight-loss treatments adequately
- Weight gain and obesity may reduce medication compliance and are thereby an important prognostic factor

Recommendations for treatment

- Basic programs for weight-gain management comprise interventions with respect to nutrition, exercise, and behavioral therapy. Weight loss programs should comprise two steps: first, weight reduction and, second, stabilization of weight
- The nutrition therapy includes several steps. Patients can enter at each step. The complete social environment should be involved. The patient should be informed about each step:
  - step 1: reduction of fat intake (possible weight loss: 3.2–4.3 kg in 6 months)
  - step 2: energy-reduced food (possible weight loss: 5.1 kg in 12 months)
  - step 3: meal replacement with formula products (possible weight loss: 6.5 kg in 3 months)
  - step 4: formula diet (possible weight loss: 0.5–2 kg in 12 weeks)
- Exercise leads to increased energy consumption. Weight loss is possible with an energy consumption of 2500 kcal/day
- Behavioral interventions can support motivation for exercise and nutrition therapy. The most important elements are:
  - self-monitoring of eating and drinking behavior and of exercise (eg, with protocols or nutrition diaries)
  - practice of flexible and controlled eating behavior
  - learning to cope with eating stimuli to reduce eating impulses
  - use of enhancement techniques (eg, praise) to support the new eating behavior and to reduce relapses
  - social support
  - management of relapse and prophylaxis

Approved medications for weight loss:

- Sibutramine: a selective serotonin and norepinephrine reuptake inhibitor that leads in the general population to weight loss of 2.8–4.4 kg in 3–12 months. Sibutramine can induce panic attacks, psychosis, or mania, and should be thereby used with caution (dosage: 5–20 mg/day)
- Orlistat: a lipase inhibitor that leads in the general population to weight loss of approximately 2.8 kg. In people with disturbed glucose tolerance, orlistat can reduce the conversion to type 2 diabetes (dosage: 120 mg three times daily with food; intake of other medication 1 hour before or after intake of orlistat)

Figure 3.27 Weight gain and obesity in schizophrenia: prevention and treatment (continues overleaf).

Weight gain and obesity in schizophrenia: prevention and treatment (continued)

Off-label medications for weight loss:

- Amantadine: originally designed for the treatment of influenza A virus. As a result of its side effects, such as depression, hallucinations, or epileptic seizures, it is currently rarely used for this indication. Two randomized controlled trials studying the effect of amantadine on weight loss in schizophrenia did not show a deterioration of the mental state (dosage: 300 mg/day, studied with olanzapine)
- Topiramate: blocks glutamate binding at the AMPA receptor and enhances the inhibitive effects of GABA receptors. It is used in epilepsy, migraine and cluster headache. Two randomized controlled trials studying the effect of topiramate on weight loss in schizophrenia did not show a deterioration of the mental state (dosage: 25–200 mg/day)
- Metformin: reduces the glucose production in the liver. Contraindications are type 1 diabetes, liver and kidney insufficiency, alcohol dependency, cardiac insufficiency (dosage: 3 × 500 mg/day)

Surgery (indicated only if other interventions have failed):

- For patients with obesity degree III (BMI ≥40 kg/m²), or obesity degree II (BMI 35–39.9 kg/m²) with severe comorbidities (eg, type 2 diabetes)

Figure 3.27 Weight gain and obesity in schizophrenia: prevention and treatment (continued). AMPA, α-amino-3-hydroxy-5-methyl-4-isoxazolepropionic acid receptor; BMI, body mass index; GABA, γ-aminobutyric acid. Adapted from Lambert [7].

Criteria for metabolic syndrome and dyslipidemia

Metabolic syndrome

Definition: three or more risk factors required for definition

Risk factors	Defining level
Abdominal obesity	Waist circumference, cm (inches)
Men	>102 (>40)
Women	>88 (>35)
Fasting plasma triglycerides (mg/dL)	≥150 or drug treatment
HDL cholesterol	Fasting HDL levels (mg/dL)
Men	<40
Women	<50

Fasting lipid levels and values for dyslipidemia (mg/dL)

	Optimal/ desirable	Near optimal	Borderline high	High/ undesirable	Very high
Total cholesterol	<200		200–239	>240	>240
LDL	<100	100–129	130–159	160–189	160–189
HDL	>60		<40		
Triglycerides	<150		150–199	200–499	200–499

Figure 3.28 Criteria for metabolic syndrome and dyslipidemia. HDL, high-density lipoprotein; LDL, low-density lipoprotein. Adapted from the National Cholesterol Education Program Expert Panel [49].

Metabolic syndrome is associated with an increased risk of developing CVD, coronary heart disease, cerebrovascular disease, and type 2 diabetes. Furthermore, there are also other CVD risk factors that are more frequent in people with schizophrenia compared with the general population, including greater prevalence of smoking (68% vs 35%), diabetes (13% vs 3%), hypertension (27% vs 17%) and lower HDL-cholesterol levels (43.7 mg/dL vs 49.3 mg/dL) [52].

The risk of weight gain, obesity, type 2 diabetes, and dyslipidemia differs considerably between different antipsychotics (Figure 3.30). Clozapine and olanzapine have a potential for causing type 2 diabetes and dyslipidemia, especially if combined with other psychotropic medications that have high weight-gain potential. Zotepine, risperidone, paliperidone, quetiapine, and amisulpride have some potential to induce

Risk factors for cardiometabolic disorders in schizophrenia, its prevalence and relative risk compared with the general population

Risk factor	Prevalence of risk factor (%)	Relative risk
Obesity	45–55	1.5–2
Smoking	50–80	2–3
Type 2 diabetes	10–14	2
Hypertension	≥18	
Dyslipidemia		≤5

Figure 3.29 Risk factors for cardiometabolic disorders in schizophrenia, its prevalence and relative risk compared with the general population. Adapted from Lambert [7].

Risk of metabolic abnormalities with different second-generation antipsychotics

Drug	Weight gain	Risk of diabetes	Worsening lipid profile
Clozapine	+++	+	+
Olanzapine	+++	+	+
Paliperidone	++	D	D
Risperidone	++	D	D
Quetiapine IR and XR	++	D	D
Aripiprazole	–	–	–
Ziprasidone	–	–	–

Figure 3.30 Risk of metabolic abnormalities with different second-generation antipsychotics. +, increased effect; –, no effect; D, discrepant results; IR, immediate release; XR, extended release. Reproduced with permission from the American Diabetes Association [53].

type 2 diabetes as these medications can induce weight gain. Ziprasidone and aripiprazole do not significantly affect body weight and are not related to type 2 diabetes and dyslipidemia (Figure 3.30). Recommendations for the prevention and management of metabolic syndrome in schizophrenia are given in Figures 3.31 and 3.32.

Antipsychotics have three main cardiovascular side effects:
- cardiac side effects, especially prolongation of the QTc interval;
- hypotension and orthostatic hypotension; and
- tachycardia.

The most common cardiac side effect of antipsychotics is the prolongation of the QTc interval. The QTc interval represents the duration of ventricular repolarization corrected by the heart rate and is usually below 400–420 ms, depending on age, gender, and time of day. A value above 500 ms is considered a clinically relevant QTc prolongation because it is associated with a higher risk of torsades de pointes and transition to ventricular fibrillation.

There is a variety of risk factors for QTc prolongation and medications known to prolong the QTc interval (Figure 3.33). The cardiovascular risks associated with various antipsychotics are summarized in Figure 3.34 and recommendations for monitoring cardiovascular side effects are listed in Figure 3.35.

Hypotension and orthostatic hypotension are related to the α-antiadrenergic effects of antipsychotics, known to occur, for example,

Monitoring protocol for patients on antipsychotic treatment							
	Baseline	4 weeks	8 weeks	12 weeks	Quarterly	Annually	Every 5 years
Personal and family history	x					x	
BMI	x	x	x	x	x		
Waist circumference	x					x	
Blood pressure	x			x		x	
Fasting plasma glucose	x			x		x	
Fasting lipid profile	x			x		x	x

Figure 3.31 **Monitoring protocol for patients on antipsychotic treatment.** BMI, body mass index. Reproduced with permission from the American Diabetes Association [53].

Recommendations for prevention and management of metabolic syndrome in schizophrenia

General recommendations

- Take responsibility for the patient with respect to psychiatric and somatic care
- Implement systematic education programs on physical diseases in schizophrenia – for students, psychiatrists, primary care physicians, patients, and relatives
- Improve parity and health-care access and provision
- Forge collaborative teamwork of psychiatrists with primary care physicians, especially in long-term outpatient treatment
- Consequent implementation of long-term treatment facilities for patients with schizophrenia, including somatic monitoring (integrated care)

General recommendations

- Consequent clinical application of already published monitoring protocols and treatment guidelines
- Preventive approach in antipsychotic treatment
- Monitoring of early warning signs for the respective physical disease (eg, weight loss, polyuria or polydipsia for diabetes)
- Regular diabetes screening (every 3 years) is indicated in patients ≥45 years or in patients with certain risk factors: (1) BMI ≥27 kg/m^2, (2) diabetes in first-degree relatives, (3) hypertension, (4) dyslipidemia (low HDL and/or low LDL values), (5) already existing metabolic syndrome, (6) women with a history of gestational diabetes, (7) positive family history for diabetes, or (8) patients with albuminuria
- Early detection of type 2 diabetes according to pathological values: (1) fasting glucose level: ≥126 mg/dL, (2) plasma glucose level: ≥200 mg/dL, HbA1c: >6.1%. Fasting glucose level of 100–126 mg/dL is classed as prediabetes
- In case of existing type 2 diabetes, refer patient to a diabetes specialist and facilitate regular (precaution) assessments
- Regular dyslipidemia screening is indicated in patients with certain risk factors: (1) BMI ≥27 kg/m^2, (2) regular imbalance between food intake and energy expenditure (mainly resting metabolism and physical activity), (3) diabetes, (4) renal insufficiency, (5) hypothyroidism, or (6) treatment with certain medications (eg, diuretics, β-blockers)
- In case of existing CVD risk factors, discuss risk–benefit ratio and possibly switch to an antipsychotic with no or low potential of weight gain (eg, aripiprazole or ziprasidone), or an antipsychotic on which the patient was successfully treated without weight gain

Figure 3.32 Recommendations for prevention and management of metabolic syndrome in schizophrenia. BMI, body mass index; CVD, cardiovascular disease; HbA1c, glycated hemoglobin; HDL, high-density lipoprotein; LDL, low-density lipoprotein. Adapted from Lambert [7].

with low-potency FGAs (eg, clozapine or quetiapine; Figure 3.34). Patients who experience hypotension must be cautioned against getting up quickly and without assistance because falls can result in injuries, particularly in elderly patients. Gradual dose titration, starting with a low dose, and monitoring of orthostatic signs minimize the risk of complications due to orthostatic hypotension.

Tachycardia is particularly relevant in patients with pre-existing cardiac disease and in patients who are treated with certain antipsychotics

Risk factors for QTc prolongation and medications that prolong QTc interval

Risk factors and patients at risk	
General risk factors	• Congenital long QT syndrome (inherited), personal history of syncope, family history of sudden death at an early age, hypokalemia, hypomagnesemia, other electrolyte imbalance, pre-existing cardiac disease or cardiovascular disease, bradycardia, female gender, older age
Patients at risk	• Individuals with severe and persistent mental illness, elderly, medically ill, overdose, concurrent drug use
Medications that can prolong QTc interval	
Antibiotics/antivirals	• Erythromycin, quinine, chloroquine, amantadine
Antiarrhythmics	• Quinidine, procainamide
Antihistamines	• Terfenadine
Antipsychotics	• Tricyclic FGAs of the phenothiazine type (eg, chlorpromazine, promethazine, perazine, thioridazine, and pimozide) • High-dose intravenous haloperidol • SGAs (eg, sertindole, ziprasidone)
Other psychotropics	• Tricyclic antidepressants • Others (eg, citalopram, chloral hydrate, lithium)
Rare or uncertain for QTc prolongation, but other cardiac problems	• Clozapine (eg, cardiomyopathy, cardiomyocarditis). Risk of myocarditis with clozapine is 1/500 to 1/10,000 treated patients. If the diagnosis is probable, clozapine should be stopped and the patient referred urgently to internal medicine

Figure 3.33 Risk factors for QTc prolongation and medications that prolong QTc interval.
FGA, first-generation antipsychotic; SGA, second-generation antipsychotic. Adapted from Lambert [7].

Risk of cardiological side effects related to second- and first-generation antipsychotics

Antipsychotic	Tachycardia	Orthostatic hypotension	QT prolongation
High-potent FGAs	(+)	(+)	(+)
Low-potent FGAs	++	+++	++
Amisulpride	0	0	(+)
Aripiprazole	0	0	(+)
Clozapine	++	+++	(+)
Olanzapine	(+)	(+)	(+)
Quetiapine	++	++	(+)
Risperidone/paliperidone	(+)	+(+)	+(+)
Ziprasidone/sertindole	(+)	(+)	+

Figure 3.34 Risk of cardiological side effects related to second- and first-generation antipsychotics. Prevalence and severity of side effects derive from the prescribing information, related research articles, and different guidelines. 0, no risk; (+), rare, possibly no difference with placebo; +, mild (lower than 1%); ++, sometimes (lower than 10%); +++, often (>10%). FGAs, first-generation antipsychotics; SGAs, second-generation antipsychotics. Adapted from Lambert [7].

Recommendations for monitoring cardiovascular side effects of antipsychotics

Risk factors and patients at risk

- ECG should be performed before initiating antipsychotic treatment in older patients and for those with the following risk factors:
  - concurrent treatment with medication that inhibits the metabolism of antipsychotics
  - concurrent treatment with medication that leads to QTc prolongation
  - positive family history for sudden death
  - syncope in the medical history
- Regular ECGs are recommended
- Risk factors should be assessed and carefully monitored (eg, diabetes, blood pressure, obesity, dyslipidemia, or previous cardiac side effects of antipsychotic treatment)
- If the QTc interval is >440 ms, medications that increase the QTc should be avoided and/or a cardiologist consulted
- If a QTc interval increases to >500 ms, the antipsychotic should be discontinued

Figure 3.35 Recommendations for monitoring cardiovascular side effects of antipsychotics. Adapted from Lambert [7].

(eg, clozapine). It is caused by the anticholinergic effects of antipsychotics but may also occur as a result of postural hypotension (see Figure 3.34).

Endocrine and sexual side effects

Assessment of potential sexual disorders should play an important role in the treatment of patients with schizophrenia. Effective assessment of sexual function disorders depends greatly on the attitude of the treating physician. However, only 6–8% of doctors reported always interviewing their patients on sexual functioning [54–56], although this aspect is important to the patients. When patients treated with antipsychotics were asked to evaluate the relative importance of 19 psychotic symptoms and 20 adverse effects, sexual dysfunction was rated the most unpleasant side effect and equally as impairing as paranoid delusions. Impotence was rated as more unpleasant than any of the psychotic symptoms [54–56].

With respect to the prevalence of sexual dysfunctions, studies reported a wide range of 30–80% with differences related to gender, type of antipsychotic treatment, type of pharmacological combination therapy, and other factors [57,58]. Female patients most often experience menstrual disorders (about 80%), of which dysmenorrhea is the most frequent. The main reported sexual disorders for male patients are ejaculation and erectile dysfunctions (30–60%) and difficulty in reaching orgasm (up to 60%; Figure 3.36) [57].

There are two main causes of sexual dysfunctions in schizophrenia: the illness itself and the pharmacological treatment. With respect to pharmacological treatment, prolactin elevation is considered to be of central importance in the etiology of sexual dysfunction. The lactotroph hormone prolactin is produced in the anterior lobe of the pituitary gland and induced physiologically by the sucking reflex. The secretion of prolactin leads to a suppression of the release of gonadotrophin. The control of prolactin synthesis and secretion is part of a complex neurochemical and

Affected persons	Short- and long-term consequences and complications
Females	• Hypogonadism (clinical manifestation of an ovarian hypofunction): − oligo-/dysmenorrhea, amenorrhea − libido dysfunctions − anovulatory cycles (infertility) − vaginal atrophy − androgenization − premenstrual syndrome with dysphoria and cognitive problems • Mastopathia, mastodynia • Galactorrhea • Vision disorders, headache • Potential increase in breast cancer risk
Males	• Hypogonadism (clinical manifestation of a testes hypofunction): − libido dysfunctions − erectile and/or ejaculatory dysfunctions − reduced spermatogenesis (oligospermia, infertility) • Gynecomastia • Galactorrhea • Vision disorders, headache
Both genders	• Skeletal system: − reduced bone mineral density caused by a long-term relative or absolute estrogen or testosterone deficiency with increased risk of osteoporosis • Cardiovascular system: − increased risk of stroke and/or arteriosclerosis • Other areas: − affective disorders (eg, depression) − cognitive dysfunctions − potential for increased risk of tardive dyskinesia
Pediatric patients (both genders)	• Delayed puberty • In males, consequences include reduced development of the skeletal muscles and disturbed bone growth • In females, consequences include infertility, reduced libido, mammary atrophy, and osteoporosis

Figure 3.36 Clinical short- and long-term consequences and complications related to increased prolactin. Adapted from Bushe et al [54], Citrome [55], and Dursun et al [56].

hormonal metabolism. The blockade of tuberoinfundibular dopamine receptors of the hypothalamus can lead to cessation of the physiological suppression of prolactin and therefore to increased prolactin levels. Besides this dopamine-mediated increase of secretion, prolactin can also be directly released through a variety of physiological and pathological mechanisms (Figure 3.37).

Normal plasma levels for both women and men are in the range 5–25 ng/mL with a high degree of interindividual variability. In a grey

The most important causes of increased prolactin

Physiological or general causes

- Pregnancy, lactation
- Acute and chronic psychological and/or physical stress
- Orgasm
- Epileptic seizure
- Intensive manipulation/sucking at the breast
- Albuminous meals and large intake of beer
- Physiological increase of prolactin in late sleep phase
- Excessive exercise

Pathological causes

- Autonomous production and secretion of prolactin
  - prolactinoma (micro- or macro-)
- Disturbed hypothalamic dopamine release or transport to the lactotroph cells of the pituitary gland
  - hypothalamic tumor (craniopharyngioma)
  - granulomatous diseases of the lining of the brain and spinal cord (eg, sarcoidosis)
  - trauma
- Stimulation of the lactotrophic adenohypophyseal cells
  - hypothyroidism
- Pharmacological medications
  - dopamine receptor antagonists (eg, some SGAs [risperidone, amisulpride, paliperidone] and FGAs [benzamide, phenothiazine, butyrophenone])
  - antihypertensive drugs (eg, reserpine)
  - monoamine synthesis inhibitors (α-methyldopa)
  - monoamine uptake inhibitors (eg, imipramine and amitriptyline)
  - serotonin reuptake inhibitors (eg, fluoxetine, sertraline, citalopram, fluvoxamine, paroxetine)
  - estrogen (in higher dosage)
  - opiates
- Other causes
  - kidney failure
  - cirrhosis of the liver
  - diseases of the leading thorax septum (eg, herpes zoster)
  - ectopic prolactin secretion
  - idiopathic functional prolactin elevation

Figure 3.37 The most important causes of increased prolactin. FGA, first-generation antipsychotics; SGA, second-generation antipsychotics. Adapted from Bushe et al [54], Citrome [55], and Dursun et al [56].

area of 25–200 ng/mL, values >40 ng/mL are related to prolactin-induced complications (Figure 3.36), and values >200 ng/mL are clearly pathological and justify an assessment of whether the patient has a tumor of the pituitary gland [7].

Different pharmacological treatments are related to a varying risk of hyperprolactinemia (Figure 3.38). The following risk order could be made from the highest to the lowest: combinations with prolactin-elevating antipsychotics > amisulpride = risperidone = paliperidone > FGAs (haloperidol) > olanzapine > quetiapine = clozapine = aripiprazole = ziprasidone.

There are several recommendations for good clinical practice regarding potential complications related to high prolactin levels (Figure 3.39):

- Patients should be educated and provided with information on this topic before initiation of antipsychotic treatment.
- Antipsychotic-related risk of hyperprolactinemia should be considered when prescribing antipsychotics.

Weighted effects of antipsychotics on prolactin levels

Antipsychotic	Prolactin response weighted score*	Hyperprolactinemia APA weighted risk[†]
Haloperidol	+++	+++
Amisulpride	+++	+++
Aripiprazole	0	0
Clozapine	+	0
Olanzapine	++/+	0
Paliperidone	ID, possibly comparable to risperidone	ID, possibly comparable to risperidone
Quetiapine IR and XR	+	0
Risperidone	+++	+++
Ziprasidone	+	+
Combination of prolactin-elevating antipsychotics	++++	++++

Figure 3.38 Weighted effects of antipsychotics on prolactin levels. *+++ = robust elevation; ++ = moderate elevation; + = mild, transient elevation; 0 = no elevation. [†]++++ = frequently causes side effect with higher prevalence and higher prolactin elevation compared with monotherapy; +++ = frequently causes side effects at therapeutic doses; + = mild or occasional side effects at therapeutic doses; 0 = no risk or rarely causes side effects at therapeutic doses. APA, American Psychiatric Association; ID, insufficient data; IR, immediate release; XR, extended release. Adapted from Lambert [7].

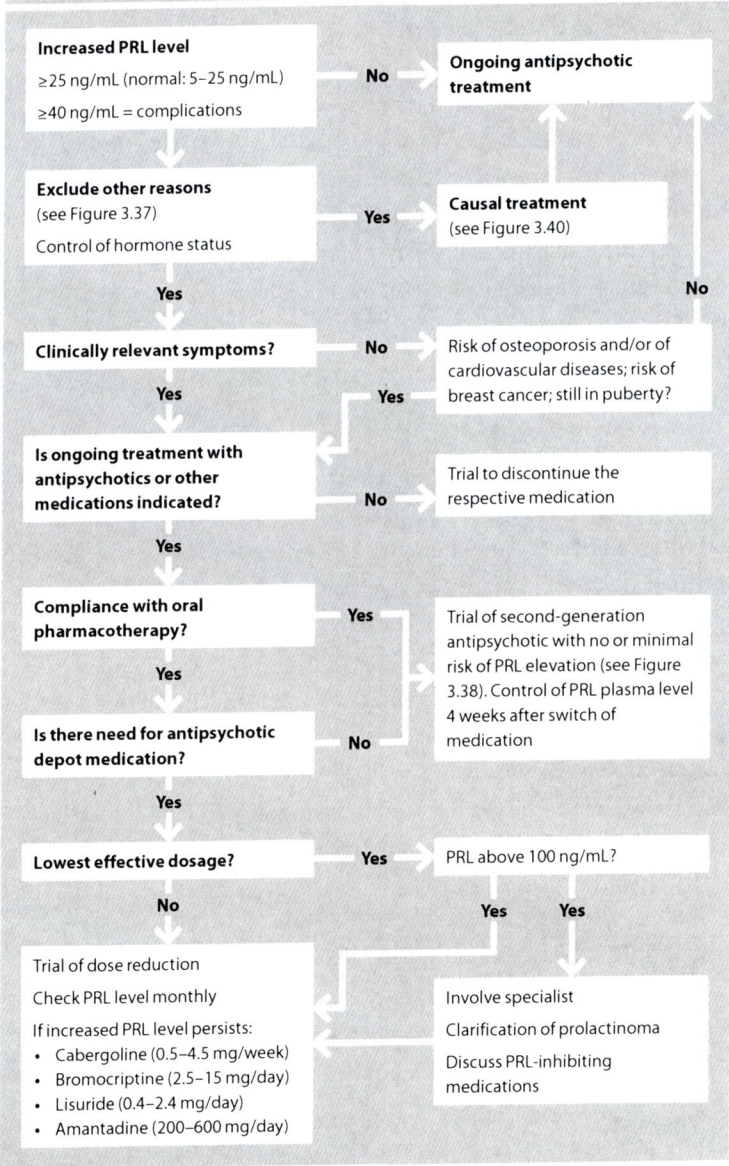

Figure 3.39 Monitoring and treatment algorithm for increased prolactin in patients with schizophrenia. PRL, prolactin. Adapted from Bushe et al [54].

- Prolactin level should be checked before start of antipsychotic treatment, and monitored throughout the treatment if the patient is treated with prolactin-elevating antipsychotics or combination therapy (see Figure 3.38).
- Patients should be regularly assessed for sexual dysfunctions and given sufficient time to talk about their sexual functioning and any impairments, because most patients try to avoid this topic.
- Treatment should follow specialized algorithms (see Figure 3.39) and, in case of chronically elevated prolactin levels, several prolactin-reducing medications could be used (Figure 3.40).

The most recommended psychosocial interventions

Eóin Killackey and Pat McGorry

In the last few years there has been a growing realization of the failure of symptomatic recovery alone to lead to functional recovery. Individuals with illness often make symptomatic recoveries due to the availability of better agents (and more evidence-based use of such agents), but are left functionally disabled, not returning to school or work and becoming socially marginalized.

For these reasons the psychosocial treatment of schizophrenia is now considered to be as important and necessary as the pharmacological treatment. This has not always been the case. Several factors prevented the inclusion of psychosocial treatments as a core part of the treatment of schizophrenia in the past. These have included the prevalent kraepelinian

Pharmacological and other treatments for increased prolactin
Causal treatment
• Operation of a prolactinoma (micro- or macro-)
• Treatment of hypothyroidism
Symptomatic treatment (normal dose to maximum dose)
• Bromocriptine: 1.25 mg twice daily oral; up to 15 mg/day
• Lisuride: 0.2 mg twice daily oral; up to 2.4 mg/day
• Cabergoline: 0.5–1.0 mg/week oral; up to 4.5 mg/week
• Amantadine: 200–300 mg/day oral; up to 600 mg/day

Figure 3.40 Pharmacological and other treatments for increased prolactin. Adapted from Bushe et al [54].

concept of dementia praecox, which posited that schizophrenia was an illness of inevitable decline, and that psychodynamic therapeutic interventions, which made up the larger part of psychosocial interventions in that era, were not effective.

General principles for use of psychosocial interventions in schizophrenia

- Psychosocial interventions should not be optional additions to treatment, but instead, wherever possible, should be part of the routine care of patients with schizophrenia.
- There is growing evidence that some of the psychosocial interventions, particularly cognitive–behavioral therapy (CBT), and vocational and family interventions, can have a major impact on the wellbeing of people with schizophrenia.
- Schizophrenia is an illness that affects people in many life domains and, as yet, medication does not address all of these deficits. Psychosocial and pharmacological interventions complement each other, and practitioners of each should work together to maximize outcomes for patients with schizophrenia.
- Patients with schizophrenia must be provided with psychosocial interventions relevant to their needs.
- When psychosocial interventions are provided, there is evidence that the quality of life and functioning of patients with schizophrenia is improved and that there is a positive effect on admission rates.
- Families feel more supported and informed and better able to look after a relative with schizophrenia when they are offered education, support, and appropriate involvement in treatment.
- Psychosocial interventions work best in a system that is not wholly occupied with managing people through the acute episodes of illness and then discharging them to minimalist care (especially primary care practitioners, where they are the sole health worker).

- The nature of the psychosocial intervention has to be tailored to the individual and should focus specifically on issues of relevance to that patient.
- Psychosocial intervention requires highly trained clinicians with expertise in specific areas (rather than a model in which these interventions are devolved to less skilled practitioners and semiskilled nongovernmental organizations).

Family interventions

Family, broadly defined as those who have an emotional and practical relationship to the person with schizophrenia (eg, parents, partner, siblings), often plays an important role in both caring for patients with schizophrenia and helping them care for themselves. However, this is a role that is often very stressful and has the potential to lead to strains on the relationships, if not to alienation. Family interventions in schizophrenia cover a wide variety of practices, which are conducted in a variety of situations. They can be: psychoeducational, therapeutic, or skill-based; conducted with or without the patient present; in multifamily groups or with one family alone; and brief in duration (eg, single or few sessions) or conducted over an extended period.

A review of 13 studies of family interventions in patients with schizophrenia found the following [59]:

- Family intervention has no effect on mortality.
- The mental state of patients improves with family therapy; however, the improvement is greater when the level of skill of the therapy team is higher.
- Drop-out rates are low, suggesting that family intervention is acceptable to patients.
- There are no clear effects in the domain of social functioning, but there are positive trends toward employment and independent living.
- The effect on families is to reduce the burden of illness, increase knowledge, and expressed emotions caused by the situation.
- Family intervention leads to cost saving, with a drop of about 20% in total costs.

- The number needed to treat to have one person symptom-free using family intervention is 6.5.
- Family therapy reduces relapse rates by over 50% compared with medication and case management alone.

Another review of six randomized controlled trials of family intervention also found that there were significant effects on relapse rates at 6 and 9 months but not 24 months, and a reported number needed to treat of between 2 and 5 [60]. There were also significant effects on expressed emotion and hospital admission but not on compliance.

Several reviews have examined studies of family intervention in schizophrenia and have reached the following conclusions:

- Family therapy is effective on a number of symptoms and is recommended.
- Family intervention should be integrated at all stages and with all aspects of care.
- Where possible, family interventions are more effective when they are more than 6 months in duration or include more than 10 planned sessions.
- Family treatment should include a psychoeducational module.
- Family intervention is effective in reducing relapse. It should be offered particularly where the family member has relapsed recently or is in danger of doing so.
- Family psychoeducational interventions are effective in reducing problems in families with difficulties.
- Multifamily groups may be better than single-family groups; however, families may have a preference for single-family groups and this should be respected where possible.
- Local and national support groups are effective in supporting the family, and referrals to patient and carer networks are recommended.

Psychoeducation programs

Psychoeducation is a process of educating the patient (and/or family) about the illness and its treatment. Psychoeducation is a necessary process enabling the patient to participate in decisions about treatment to the fullest degree possible. There have been a number of positive results with psychoeducation programs in patients with schizophrenia. These include improved adherence to treatment, better outcomes, better management of subsequent relapse, lower readmission rates, and a positive effect on patients' wellbeing.

Psychoeducation can be conducted separately, but it can also be included as a part of other interventions, such as family intervention (see above). Psychoeducation in the early phases tends to focus on supporting and educating the individual or family about schizophrenia, generally from a biopsychosocial perspective. As the patient progresses in his or her recovery, the subject matter may change to more general topics, such as life skills and adapting to the changes necessary to manage the illness.

Information should also be given to other people who may not be primary carers, but who frequently come into contact with patients with schizophrenia. These may include workers at community agencies, local government employees, and workers at supported accommodation residences, as well as the general public. The term for this process is mental health literacy rather than psychoeducation.

A Cochrane review of psychoeducation for patients with schizophrenia found that, compared with standard care alone, the addition of psychoeducation made a worthwhile contribution. A NICE review found that, although it is good practice to provide psychoeducation, there is not yet enough evidence of its effect on outcome to recommend it as a discrete treatment. Thus, in summary:

- Psychoeducation for patients possibly reduces relapse, through improved compliance. It also increases patient satisfaction with treatment and improves their knowledge of schizophrenia.
- However, the evidence of its ability to reduce relapse is not yet conclusive enough to recommend its use as a discrete intervention.
- Psychoeducation for families is also effective and should be offered routinely.

Cognitive interventions

Although Aaron Beck used cognitive therapy techniques to treat psychotic symptoms in at least one patient in the early 1950s, the development of further work in this area began in earnest only after the reconceptualization of schizophrenia from a single syndrome to a cluster of separate symptoms, each of which varied and could be addressed individually. There are two strategies in the cognitive interventions: one is what may be called the CBT strategy, which seeks to use the techniques of CBT to reduce distress and symptoms; the second strategy is cognitive remediation, which directly addresses the cognitive deficits that are evident in patients with schizophrenia. Both of these strategies are described in more detail in this section.

Cognitive–behavioral therapy interventions

CBT interventions involve the therapist and patient exploring the links between thoughts (which may be delusional) and feelings. The therapist may challenge the validity of some thoughts and perceptions, testing them against other possible hypotheses that could explain the experience. It has been reported that CBT in combination with standard care was better at reducing relapse compared with standard care alone. Furthermore, for CBT to be effective, those who administer it need to be skilled in its application.

A review conducted in the preparation of the NICE guidelines found that CBT intervention had better effects when the intervention lasted for more than 6 months or had at least 10 planned sessions. It also found that CBT intervention showed good efficacy with those who had persistent psychotic symptoms [61]. Recommendations for CBT are given in Figure 3.41.

Recommendations for use of cognitive–behavioral therapy in schizophrenia

- Individual CBT is highly effective in improving the mental state and global functioning of a patient, as it is associated with reduced risk of relapse compared to standard care alone
- CBT in the acute phase can accelerate recovery and hasten discharge when added to standard care
- CBT can be helpful in reducing symptoms of treatment-resistant schizophrenia
- CBT should be offered particularly to those who have persistent symptoms
- CBT should be available to all people with schizophrenia
- CBT is an intervention that requires a skilled practitioner

Figure 3.41 Recommendations for use of cognitive–behavioral therapy in schizophrenia. CBT, cognitive–behavioral therapy.

Cognitive remediation

Another cognitive intervention used in the treatment of schizophrenia is cognitive remediation (sometimes known as cognitive rehabilitation). The aim of cognitive remediation is to address cognitive impairments of patients with schizophrenia (eg, distractibility, memory problems, lack of vigilance, attentional deficits, and limitations in planning and decision-making). It is hoped that, by addressing these issues, patients will be more able to take advantage of other interventions and better able to function in social and other domains. So far, results in controlled trials of cognitive remediation have been equivocal. Consequently, the NICE guidelines, along with other international guidelines, have concluded that at present there is not enough evidence to recommend cognitive remediation as an evidence-based intervention.

Social-skills training

Schizophrenia most commonly occurs for the first time in young people (children, adolescents, and young adults) and, as a result, patients with schizophrenia often do not engage in many of the normal developmental tasks of late adolescence and early adulthood. These tasks include developing social skills, intimate relationships, occupational skills, and independent living skills. In addition, those who develop schizophrenia later in life often acquire deficits in these areas. Social-skills training (also called "life-skills training") is a widely practiced intervention and seeks to address these deficits.

Evidence shows that social-skills training improves social adjustment, enlarges or enhances the social network of the patient, and contributes significantly to the development of independent living skills. A 1997 report claimed that a small number of studies had shown that skills taught in programs tend to be general and do not address specific individual needs, although more research is needed in this area. Both the Cochrane and NICE reviews of social-skills training found no evidence to support its benefit, although it has been demonstrated in a number of independent studies. However, NICE guidelines suggest that social and physical activities should be a required part of the care plan for all patients with schizophrenia [1]. There is, therefore, a need for well-planned and conducted studies to examine the effectiveness of social-skills training.

Vocational rehabilitation

One of the associated features of schizophrenia is low socioeconomic status. In high-income societies, unemployment rate among severely mentally ill patients is estimated at 70–90% [62]. Apart from being a fundamental right, being employed in a paid or voluntary capacity can have a clinical impact by increasing self-esteem, alleviating psychiatric symptoms, and reducing dependency and relapse. An intervention that aims to address the issue of employment for patients with schizophrenia is vocational rehabilitation.

Sheltered workshops were the original vocational rehabilitation model. However, these did not lead to many people getting competitive employment. At present, there are two main models of vocational rehabilitation: prevocational training, in which a period of preparation is engaged in before seeking competitive employment; and supported employment, in which people are placed in competitive employment with the provision of on-the-job support. Cochrane review of vocational rehabilitation found that supported employment was a more effective program than prevocational training. A total of 34% of people engaged in the supported employment program were still working at 12 months compared with 12% in the prevocational training conditions. The most well-defined form of supported employment is known as individual placement and support, an evidenced-based, practice-supported employment initiative that coordinates mental health services and employment services to assist in rapid job placement tailored to an individual's interests and skills. There is emerging evidence that early intervention in the vocational domain using individual placement and support for young people with a first-episode illness leads to even better outcomes than later interventions.

Based on these findings, patients with schizophrenia should be encouraged, where possible, to find a meaningful occupation in either a paid or a voluntary capacity. In addition, patients with schizophrenia should be put in contact with agencies that provide such services early in the course of illness:

- Becoming vocationally involved is likely to have positive psychosocial consequences.
- People with mental illnesses, including those with schizophrenia, want to find work, but, at present, there is an extremely disproportionate number of patients with mental illnesses who are unemployed.
- Various models of vocational rehabilitation have had different levels of success in placing people in competitive positions.
- Supported employment programs are much more successful than other types of programs.
- Vocational rehabilitation programs can reduce rehospitalization and improve insight.
- Vocational rehabilitation enhances vocational functioning.

Compliance therapy

One of the problems that clinicians working with people with schizophrenia are faced with is the issue of treatment compliance (Chapter 2, page 27). There are many reasons why patients are not compliant. Overall, it is often difficult to adjust to regularly taking medicine (which often has unpleasant side effects), especially when this lifestyle change is combined with amotivation and low insight that often accompany schizophrenia. Compliance therapy has been developed that specifically addresses the issue of compliance and focuses on educating the patient on the link between compliance and a favorable outcome.

Compliance therapy uses motivational interviewing and cognitive–behavioral techniques to help clients explore issues around compliance. It may be useful when applied in both early and later phases of recovery. Compliance therapy has been found to be effective in increasing compliance with treatment in one randomized controlled trial, and further research is needed to confirm the validity of this intervention.

Summary of psychosocial interventions

The most important recommendations for the use of psychosocial interventions are given in Figure 3.42. After decades of receiving little, if any,

Recommendations for use of psychosocial interventions in schizophrenia

- Can address a range of important domains not always addressed by medication
- Have a positive impact on the quality of life of patients with schizophrenia and their carers
- Where possible should be offered as part of a package that has a pharmacotherapeutic basis but includes some or all of:
  - psychological therapy (CBT)
  - vocational interventions
  - family interventions
  - psychoeducation
  - compliance therapy
- Must be administered by people trained in their application

Figure 3.42 Recommendations for use of psychosocial interventions in schizophrenia.
CBT, cognitive–behavioral therapy.

consideration, psychosocial interventions are making a comeback and are being viewed as a necessary complement to the ever-advancing sophistication of pharmacotherapy. Some interventions, such as CBT, vocational rehabilitation, and family interventions, already have a good deal of evidence to support them; others are now being tested.

Increasingly, the role of managing patients with schizophrenia is being devolved to primary care doctors in many countries around the world. It is important, therefore, that doctors make themselves aware of the psychosocial interventions that are evidence-based and available in their area. Where there are no such services, doctor and patient groups should use the available evidence to lobby for the provision of such services.

References

1   The 2009 National Institute for Health and Clinical Excellence guideline on core interventions in the treatment and management of schizophrenia in adults in primary and secondary care (updated edition). The National Institute for Health and Clinical Excellence website. www.nice.org.uk/guidance/CG82/NICEGuidance. Accessed April 2, 2012.

2   American Psychiatric Association. Practice Guideline for the Treatment of Patients with Schizophrenia, 2nd compendium. Arlington, VA: APA, 2004.

3   Kreyenbuhl J, Buchanan RW, Dickerson FB, Dixon LB; Schizophrenia Patient Outcomes Research Team (PORT). The Schizophrenia Patient Outcomes Research Team (PORT): updated treatment recommendations 2009. Schizophr Bull. 2010;36:94-103.

4   Canadian Psychiatric Association. Clinical practice guidelines. Treatment of schizophrenia. Can J Psychiatry. 2005;50(13 suppl 1):7S-57S.

5   Royal Australian and New Zealand College of Psychiatrists Clinical Practice Guidelines Team for the Treatment of Schizophrenia and Related Disorders. Royal Australian and New Zealand College of Psychiatrists clinical practice guidelines for the treatment of schizophrenia and related disorders. Aust N Z J Psychiatry. 2005;39:1-30.

6 Weiden PJ, Preskorn SH, Fahnestock PA, Carpenter D, Ross R, Docherty JP. Translating the psychopharmacology of antipsychotics to individualized treatment for severe mental illness: a roadmap. *J Clin Psychiatry*. 2007;68(suppl 7):1-48.

7 Lambert M. *Taschenatlas der Pharmakotherapie psychotischer Störungen*. Stuttgart, Germany: Thieme-Verlag, 2009.

8 Nielsen J, Damkier P, Lublin H, Taylor D. Optimizing clozapine treatment. *Acta Psychiatr Scand*. 2011;123:411-422.

9 Potkin SG, Bera R, Gulasekaram B, et al. Plasma clozapine concentrations predict clinical response in treatment-resistant schizophrenia. *J Clin Psychiatry*. 1994;55(suppl B):133-136.

10 The International Psychopharmacology Algorithm Project schizophrenia algorithm. The International Psychopharmacology Algorithm Project website. www.ipap.org/pdf/schiz/IPAP_Schiz_flowchart20060327.pdf. Accessed April 2, 2012.

11 Huber CG, Naber D, Lambert M. Incomplete remission and treatment resistance in first-episode psychosis: definition, prevalence and predictors. *Expert Opin Pharmacother*. 2008;12:2027-2038.

12 Lambert M, Naber D, Huber CG. Management of incomplete remission and treatment resistance in first-episode psychosis. *Expert Opin Pharmacother*. 2008;9:2039-2051.

13 Bruch SM, Zeller S. Agitation I: overview of agitation and violence. In: Glick RL, Berlin JS, Fishkind AB, Zeller SL, eds. *Emergency Psychiatry: Principles and Practice*. Philadelphia, PA: Lippincott Williams & Wilkins; 2008:117-124.

14 Allen MH, Currier GW, Carpenter D, et al. Treatment of behavioral emergencies. *J Psychiatr Pract*. 2005;11:5-108.

15 Lambert M, Naber D, eds. *Current Schizophrenia*. 2nd edn. New York, NY: Springer Healthcare; 2009.

16 Stroup TS, Marder SR, Lieberman JA. Pharmacotherapies. In: Lieberman JA, Stroup TS, Perkins DO, eds. *Essential Schizophrenia*. Arlington, VA: American Psychiatric Publishing, Inc.; 2012:173-206.

17 Haldol [package insert]. Titusville, NJ: Ortho-McNeil Neurologics; 2011.

18 Zyprexa [package insert]. Indianapolis, IN: Eli Lilly and Company; 2011.

19 Geodon [package insert].New York, NY: Roerig; 2010.

20 Nemeroff CB, Lieberman JA, Weiden PJ, et al. From clinical research to clinical practice: a 4-year review of ziprasidone.*CNS Spectr*. 2005;10(suppl 17):1-20.

21 Fitzgerald P. Long-acting antipsychotic medication, restraint and treatment in the management of acute psychosis. *Aust N Z J Psychiatry*. 1999;33:660-666.

22 Cookson J, Taylor D, Katona C. Violence: assessing risk and acute tranquilisation. In: *Use of Drugs in Psychiatry*. 5th edn. London, England: The Royal College of Psychiatrists; 2002:154-162.

23 Addington D, Bouchard R-H, Goldberg J, et al. Clinical practice guidelines: treatment of schizophrenia. *Can J Psychiatry*. 2005;50(suppl 1):1S-56S.

24 Droperidol injection [package insert]. Shirley, NY: American Regent, Inc.; 2009.

25 Clozaril [package insert]. East Hanover, NJ: Novartis Pharmaceuticals Corporation; 2011.

26 Kerwin RW, Bolonna A. Management of clozapine-resistant schizophrenia. *Adv Psychiatr Treat*. 2005;11:101-106.

27 Remington G, Saha A, Chong S-A, Shammi C. Augmentation strategies in clozapine-resistant schizophrenia. *CNS Drugs*. 2005;19:843-872.

28 Nasrallah HA, Tandon R. Classic antipsychotic medications. In: Schatzberg AF, Nemeroff CB, eds. *The American Psychiatric Publishing Textbook of Psychopharmacology*. 4th ed. Arlington, VA: American Psychiatric Publishing, Inc.; 2009:533-554.

29 Dev VJ, Rosenberg T, Krupp P. Agranulocytosis and clozapine. *BMJ*. 1994;309:54.

30 Davis, JM, Kane JM, Marder SR, et al. Dose response of prophylactic antipsychotics. *J Clin Psych*. 1993;54(suppl):24-30.

31 Anderson CM, Reiss DJ, Hogarty GE. *Schizophrenia and the Family: A Practitioner's Guide to Psychoeducation and Management*. New York, NY: The Guilford Press; 1986.

32 Kane JM. Treatment programme and long-term outcome in chronic schizophrenia. *Acta Psychiatr Scand*. 1990;82(suppl 358):151-157.

33 Robinson D, Woerner MG, Alvir JM, et al. Predictors of relapse following response from a first episode of schizophrenia or schizoaffective disorder. *Arch Gen Psychiatry*. 1999;56:241-247.

34 Wyatt RJ. Research in schizophrenia and the discontinuation of antipsychotic medications. *Schizophr Bull*. 1997;23:3-9.

35 Bakker PR, de Groot IW, van Os J, van Harten PN. Long-stay psychiatric patients: a prospective study revealing persistent antipsychotic-induced movement disorder. *PLoS One*. 2011;6:e25588.

36 Halliday J, Farrington S, Macdonald S, MacEwan T, Sharkey V, McCreadie R. Nithsdale Schizophrenia Surveys 23: movement disorders. 20-year review. *Br J Psychiatry*. 2002;181:422-427.

37 Schooler NR, Kane JM. Research diagnoses for tardive dyskinesia. *Arch Gen Psychiatry*. 1982;39:486-487.

38 Correll CU, Schenk EM. Tardive dyskinesia and new antipsychotics. *Curr Opin Psychiatry*. 2008;21:151-156.

39 Tenback DE, van Harten PN. Epidemiology and risk factors for (tardive) dyskinesia. *Int Rev Neurobiol*. 2011;98:211-230.

40 Gillman PK. Neuroleptic malignant syndrome: mechanisms, interactions, and causality. *Mov Disord*. 2010;25:1780-1790.

41 Strawn JR, Keck PE Jr, Caroff SN. Neuroleptic malignant syndrome. *Am J Psychiatry*. 2007 Jun;164:870-876.

42 Ananth J, Parameswaran S, Gunatilake S, Burgoyne K, Sidhom T. Neuroleptic malignant syndrome and atypical antipsychotic drugs. *J Clin Psychiatry*. 2004;65:464-470.

43 Pelonero AL, Levenson JL, Pandurangi AK.. Neuroleptic malignant syndrome: a review. *Psychiatr Serv*. 1998;49:1163-1172.

44 De Hert M, Schreurs V, Vancampfort D, van Winkel R. Metabolic syndrome in people with schizophrenia: a review. *World Psychiatry*. 2009;8:15-22.

45 National Institutes of Health. Clinical guidelines on the identification, evaluation, and treatment of overweight and obesity in adults – the evidence report. *Obes Res*. 1998;6(suppl 2):51S-209S.

46 Zipursky RB, Gu H, Green AI, Perkins DO, et al. Course and predictors of weight gain in people with first-episode psychosis treated with olanzapine or haloperidol. *Br J Psychiatry*. 2005;187:537-543.

47 Hummer M, Kemmler G, Kurz M, Kurzthaler I, Oberbauer H, Fleischhacker WW. Weight gain induced by clozapine. *Eur Neuropsychopharmacol*. 1995;5:437-440.

48 Newcomer JW, Haupt DW. The metabolic effects of antipsychotic medications. *Can J Psychiatry*. 2006;51:480-491.

49 Detection, evaluation, and treatment of high blood cholesterol in adults (Adult Treatment Panel III). National Institutes of Health website. www.nhlbi.nih.gov/guidelines/cholesterol/atp3xsum.pdf. Accesed April 2, 2012.

50 De Hert M, van Winkel R, Van Eyck D, et al. Prevalence of diabetes, metabolic syndrome and metabolic abnormalities in schizophrenia over the course of the illness: a cross-sectional study. *Clin Pract Epidemiol Ment Health*. 2006;2:14-26.

51 McEvoy JP, Meyer JM, Goff DC, et al. Prevalence of the metabolic syndrome in patients with schizophrenia: baseline results from the Clinical Antipsychotic Trials of Intervention Effectiveness (CATIE) schizophrenia trial and comparison with national estimates from NHANES III. *Schizophr Res*. 2005;80:19-32.

52 Goff DC, Sullivan LM, McEvoy JP, et al. A comparison of ten-year cardiac risk estimates in schizophrenia patients from the CATIE study and matched controls. *Schizophr Res*. 2005;80:45-53.

53 American Diabetes Association; American Psychiatric Association; American Association of Clinical Endocrinologists; North American Association for the Study of Obesity. Consensus development conference on antipsychotic drugs and obesity and diabetes. *J Clin Psychiatry*. 2004;65:267-272.

54 Bushe C, Shaw M, Peveler RC. A review of the association between antipsychotic use and hyperprolactinaemia. *J Psychopharmacol*. 2008;22:46-55.

55 Citrome L. Current guidelines and their recommendations for prolactin monitoring in psychosis. *J Psychopharmacol*. 2008;22:90-97.

56 Dursun SM, Wildgust HJ, Strickland P, Goodwin GM, Citrome L, Lean M. The emerging physical health challenges of antipsychotic associated hyperprolactinaemia in patients with serious mental illness. *J Psychopharmacol*. 2008;22:3-5.

57 Cutler AJ. Sexual dysfunction and antipsychotic treatment. *Psychoneuroendocrinology*. 2003;28 (suppl 1):69-82.

58 Hellewell, JSE. Tolerability and patient satisfaction as determinants of treatment choice in schizophrenia: a multi-national survey of the attitudes and perceptions of psychiatrists towards novel and conventional antipsychotics. Poster presented at: 13th European College of Neuropsychopharmacology Congress; September 9-13, 2000; Munich, Germany.

59 Pharoah F, Mari J, Rathbone J, Wong W. Family intervention for schizophrenia. *Cochrane Database Syst Rev*. 2010(12): CD000088.

60 Mari JJ, Streiner DL. An overview of family interventions and relapse on schizophrenia: meta-analysis of research findings. *Psychol Med*. 1994;24:565-578.

61 Turkington D, Kingdon D, Weiden PJ. Cognitive behavior therapy for schizophrenia. Am J Psychiatry. 2006;163:365-373.

62 World Health Organization. *Mental Health and Work: Impact, Issues and Good Practices*. Geneva, Switzerland: World Health Organization; 2000.

Chapter 4

Quick reference

Martin Lambert and Dieter Naber

Epidemiology, etiology, and course of illness

Epidemiology

Prevalence

The mean incidence of schizophrenia reported in epidemiological studies, when the diagnosis is limited to core criteria and corrected for age, is 15.2 per 100,000 (range 7.7–43.0 per 100,00) [1]. Average rates for men and women are 1.4 to 1, although the mean age of onset is about 5 years greater in women (hence a lower female rate in adolescence), with a second smaller peak after the menopause. The median 1-year prevalence is 3.3 per 1000, the median lifetime prevalence is 4.0 per 1000, and the mean lifetime morbidity risk is 11.3 per 1000. The latter is concurrent with the 1% risk cited in literature. However, the median lifetime morbidity risk is 7.2 per 1000 and thereby lower than 1% [2]. Services with the capacity for early detection have reported even higher annual rates of 16.7 per 10,000 in men and 8.1 per 10,000 in women among 15- to 19-year-old individuals [3].

Age at onset

Childhood onset (defined as onset by the age of 12 years) is rare: up to 1% of all schizophrenia spectrum disorders manifest before the age of 10 years, 5% before the age of 15 years, and almost 20% before the age of 18 years [4]. In most cases (30–40%), onset is in early adulthood, at the age of 18–25 years [5]. However, some people experience a later onset:

M. Lambert and D. Naber, *Current Schizophrenia*,
DOI: 10.1007/978-1-908517-68-5_4,
© Springer Healthcare, a part of Springer Science+Business Media 2012

so-called late-onset schizophrenia (patients aged >40 years) and very-late-onset schizophrenia-like psychosis (onset after the age of 60 years) [6].

Gender differences

The lifetime risk for schizophrenia seems to be equal in both sexes. It was previously reported that women tend to have a later age of onset (by 3–4 years) and a second peak of onset around the menopause [7]. However, newer epidemiologic studies with early detection have not found gender differences with respect to age at onset. Although, it is possible that women experience a more benign course of illness, especially in the short term, with better premorbid functioning, including social and intellectual abilities, more affective and less negative symptoms, and lower rates of comorbid substance abuse. In addition, a higher risk of schizophrenia has been described in women with a positive family history of psychosis than in men.

Etiology

Overview

Evidence suggests that schizophrenia is probably not related to a single biologic defect. Rather, an interaction of different pathologic mechanisms, including intrinsic and extrinsic risk factors, is more likely. These risk and/or premorbid factors may be associated with an increased vulnerability for schizophrenia. The relationships between risk factors and the diagnosis and course of schizophrenia are not fully assessed, and many questions remain unanswered about the diagnostic specificity and etiological significance of these associations. Risk factors are shown in Figure 4.1 and include, among others:
- an illness that is combined with severe central nervous system dysfunctions (eg, multiple sclerosis);
- central nervous system dysfunctions caused by various substances (eg, amphetamine psychosis);
- genetic predisposition (eg, positive family history of psychosis);
- intrauterine and/or birth complications (eg, viral infections or hypoxia);
- certain patterns of family interaction and life events; and
- extrinsic factors, such as substance abuse or developmental stress.

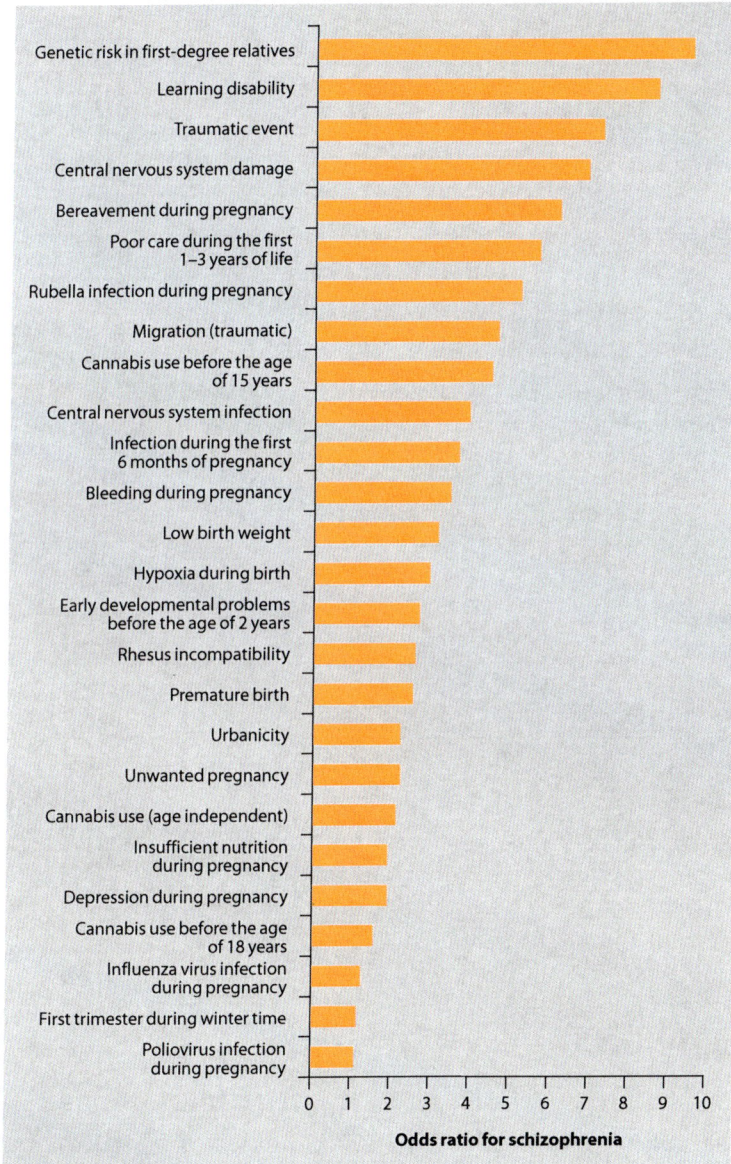

Figure 4.1 Risk factors for the development of schizophrenia. Note that these risk factors were explored and assessed in different studies with varying methodologies. As such, it is not possible to compare the sizes of the shown odds ratios. Adapted from Lambert [8].

Most of these risk factors may operate very early in life (eg, during the perinatal period), creating a disruption in the brain development followed by an increased vulnerability for stress (eg, environmental stress, toxins, or neuronal dysfunction and damage). It seems to be clear that environmental factors both add to and interact with genetic factors to produce the onset of the clinical disorder.

Genetic findings

Repeated studies of families, twins, and adopted individuals have demonstrated that genetic factors are of major relevance in schizophrenia (Figure 4.2). Lifetime prevalence differs markedly between relatives of those with and without schizophrenia (0.5–16% vs 0.2–2%) [8]. Children of a parent diagnosed with schizophrenia have a tenfold increased risk

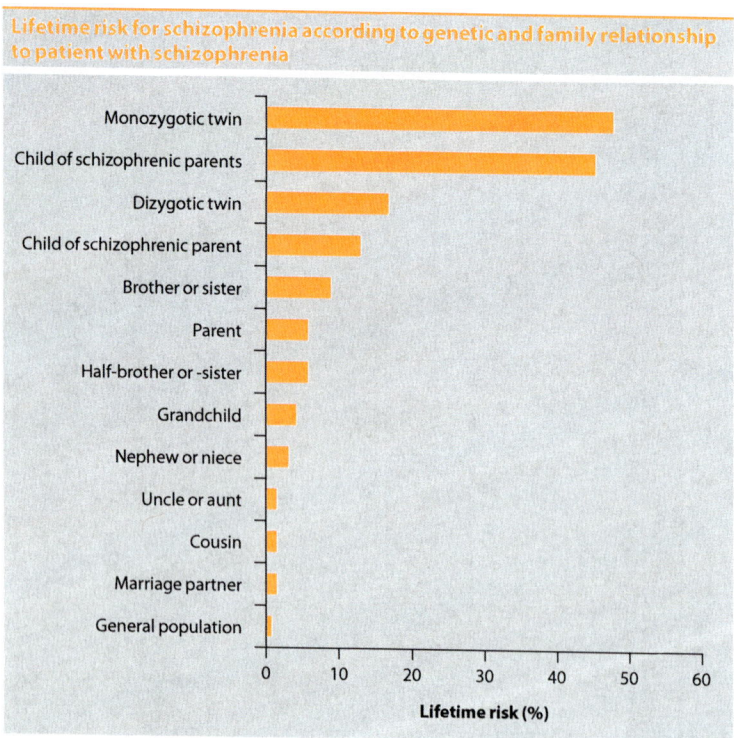

Figure 4.2 **Lifetime risk for schizophrenia according to genetic and family relationship to patient with schizophrenia.** Adapted from Lambert [8].

of developing the disorder [9]. Studies of twins suggest the importance of genetic factors, demonstrating higher rates of concordance for the disorder in monozygotic twins (44.3%) than in dizygotic twins (12.1%), proved by consistent ratios across the studies [10]. Analyses of adopted individuals provide further evidence for genetic vulnerability, showing an association between biological relatives separated at birth (tenfold increased risk) [11]. Moreover, schizophrenia spectrum disorders have a significant familial relationship with schizophrenia [12].

Structural and functional brain abnormalities

There is a large body of evidence that indicates that people with schizophrenia display abnormalities in electroencephalography, computed tomography, magnetic resonance imaging, positron emission tomography scanning, eye tracking, neurologic signs, cognitive impairment, and psychophysiology. However, the mechanisms of the associations are not known. There is no singular pathology or laboratory test to confirm the presence of schizophrenia.

Course of illness

Prodromal phase

A prodrome in schizophrenia could be defined as:

- the earliest form of psychosis; and
- a syndrome conferring increased vulnerability to psychosis.

Most of these symptoms are not specific for psychosis and also exist in other psychiatric disorders. Usually, they are subtle, self-experienced disturbances of affect and cognition, possibly accompanied by unusual perceptions. The duration of the prodromal phase can be extremely variable and its onset and separation from the phase of duration of untreated psychosis or nonpsychotic psychiatric disorders may be difficult. Common prodromal changes could be separated into symptomatic and behavioral deteriorations. Results of various studies underline the hope that early detection can help to identify people with a vulnerability to the development of psychosis or schizophrenia. These studies conclude that the rates of transition from normal or prodrome to psychosis are 33–58% in a time frame of up to 12 months [13]. However, even though these findings are encouraging, caution must be taken to avoid stigmatization and false-positive interventions.

Duration of untreated psychosis

For patients first presenting with schizophrenia, the duration of untreated psychosis (DUP; time between the onset of positive psychotic symptoms and the initiation of treatment) and the duration of untreated illness (DUI; time between onset of first prodromal symptoms and the initiation of treatment) vary widely, from a few weeks to several years. Measured in different countries, DUP ranges between 1 and 2 years [14]. Risk factors for delayed initial treatment include denial of illness, self-withdrawal from social networks, negative psychopathology, young age at onset, poor premorbid functioning, and poor insight into self-care and treatment. Some studies report a significant inverse negative correlation between long DUP or long DUI and symptomatic outcome; others have not found this correlation. Other psychosocial variables have shown a negative association with a longer phase of active psychosis. Early detection can help to reduce DUP and influence patient prognosis positively at initial treatment.

Psychotic acute phase

Negative symptoms occur as the initial psychopathology in 70% of the cases of schizophrenia [15]; mixed negative and positive symptoms occur in 20%; and only positive symptoms are observed in 10% [8]. The initial psychopathologic syndrome includes combined delusions and hallucinations in 43% of patients; undifferentiated symptoms occur in 30% of patients; and negative symptoms are observed in 13% of patients [8]. In approximately 70% of patients the illness starts slowly and chronically, with only 15–20% starting with an acute episode [8]. Delusions are reported to be the most common initial psychotic symptoms (in up to 50%), followed by hallucinations (in up to 30%) [8]. Besides psychotic symptoms, many patients with schizophrenia demonstrate cognitive impairments already evident before the initial treatment (see Chapter 2, page 19).

Agitation is another frequent problem in the acute phase of schizophrenia that is often combined with violent and destructive behavior, personal distress and suffering, self-harm, and harm to caregivers and others (see Chapter 3, page 93). Researchers who studied the consequences of agitation found that [16]:

- an average of eight assaults per year occur in a typical psychiatric service;
- mechanic restraints are used in 8.5% of patients with a mean duration of 3.3 ± 2.9 hours; and
- approximately 50–150 deaths per year occur in the context of physical restraints.

However, these rates may vary across mental health systems and services.

Psychiatric comorbidity is also frequent in schizophrenia. Approximately 80–90% of patients with schizophrenia have at least one comorbid psychiatric condition [17]. This has negative consequences for prognosis and contributes to the high rate of morbidity and mortality. Depression is associated with suicide, one of the leading causes of premature death in patients with schizophrenia [18]. Also, substance abuse disorders are associated with poor outcome (up to 70% of patients, depending on the availability of drugs) [17]. Other relevant comorbid psychiatric disorders are post-traumatic stress disorder, panic and anxiety disorders, obsessive–compulsive disorder, and social phobias, all of which may worsen prognosis. Moreover, comorbid medical conditions, including cardiac and pulmonary disease, infectious diseases, diabetes, hyperlipidemia, hypogonadism, and osteoporosis are not often sufficiently recognized and are undertreated.

Long-term phase and outcome

In many cases schizophrenia is a long-term illness with persistent symptoms and impairment of role functioning. According to one study, symptomatic evolution data show that 22% of patients who have one episode of schizophrenia do not experience long-term disability, and 35% of those who have repeated episodes do so without disability. Approximately 8% of patients have repeated episodes with stable disability, and 35% have several episodes with increasing long-term disability [19]. It was also shown that, in a 23-year follow-up period in one study, only 9% of the patients had a single psychotic episode, 32% were found to experience two or three episodes, and 36% had four or more episodes. Long-term hospitalization was required for 24% of the patients. The average number of episodes in the 23-year assessment period was 3.5 [20].

In the long term, episodes with predominant positive symptoms decrease, whereas episodes with negative symptoms increase. Symptoms, such as delusions or hallucinations, may persist, but they become attenuated over the course of the illness. Repeated episodes can be triggered by several factors, mainly comorbidity, medication noncompliance, and life events. On average, 10–20% of patients with schizophrenia have a positive outcome, and 40–50% have a negative outcome in a follow-up period of 40 years from the first episode [21]. Full remission without any disability is rare, with only 10–20% of patients showing complete remission in 5 years, and 7% in 25 years [22]. However, this course can be tempered greatly by the degree and quality of intervention provided.

Presentations and diagnosis

Clinical presentation

Schizophrenia is probably one of the most complex psychiatric disorders. Even in the early stages of the disorder (eg, prodromal phase or first episode) many patients present with a variety of different symptoms, comorbid psychiatric and somatic disorders, and interrelated social and psychologic dysfunctions (Figure 4.3).

Patients usually present with positive, negative, and disorganized symptoms (Figures 4.3 and 4.4):

- Positive symptoms include, most importantly, hallucinations (false perceptions in any of the senses) and delusions (false beliefs held with great certainty, preoccupying the individual's mind, which are socioculturally inappropriate).
- Negative symptoms typically include the reduction of social and/or personal interests, anhedonia, blunted or inappropriate emotions, and inactivity. People with schizophrenia often display negative symptoms long before the first positive symptoms emerge and, in the long term, so-called residual symptoms.
- Disorganized symptoms include disorganized thought, speech, and behavior.

Symptoms, comorbid psychiatric symptoms and disorders, and resulting psychosocial dysfunctions in patients with schizophrenia

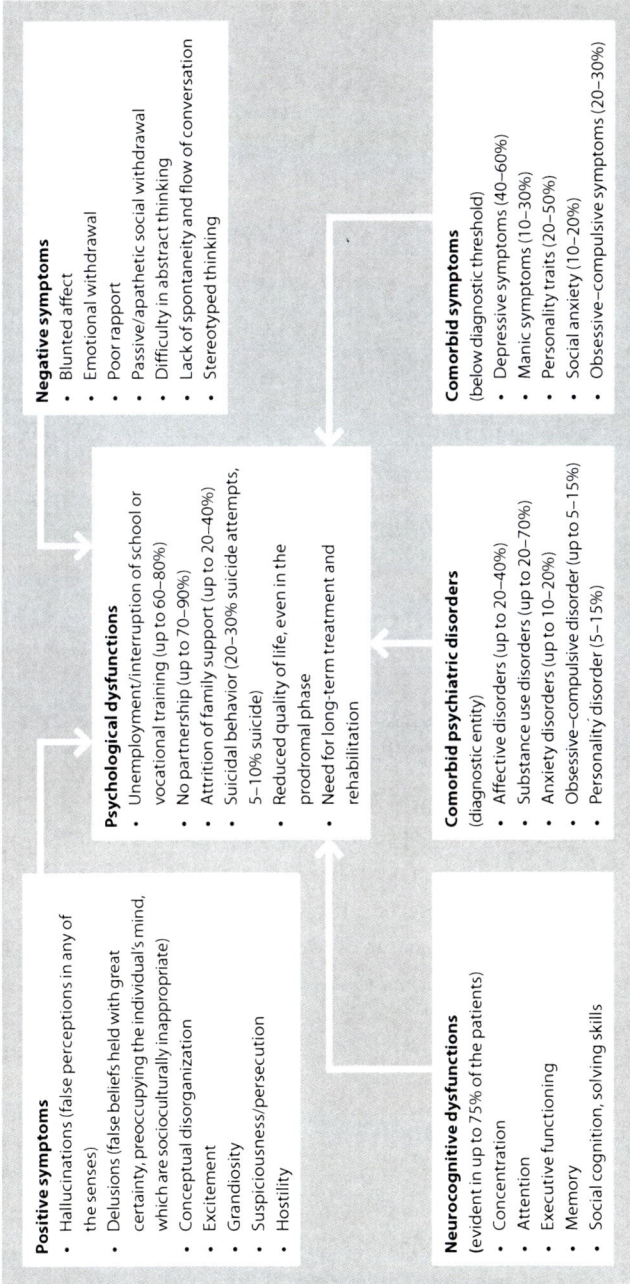

Positive symptoms

- Hallucinations (false perceptions in any of the senses)
- Delusions (false beliefs held with great certainty, preoccupying the individual's mind, which are socioculturally inappropriate)
- Conceptual disorganization
- Excitement
- Grandiosity
- Suspiciousness/persecution
- Hostility

Neurocognitive dysfunctions
(evident in up to 75% of the patients)

- Concentration
- Attention
- Executive functioning
- Memory
- Social cognition, solving skills

Psychological dysfunctions

- Unemployment/interruption of school or vocational training (up to 60–80%)
- No partnership (up to 70–90%)
- Attrition of family support (up to 20–40%)
- Suicidal behavior (20–30% suicide attempts, 5–10% suicide)
- Reduced quality of life, even in the prodromal phase
- Need for long-term treatment and rehabilitation

Comorbid psychiatric disorders
(diagnostic entity)

- Affective disorders (up to 20–40%)
- Substance use disorders (up to 20–70%)
- Anxiety disorders (up to 10–20%)
- Obsessive–compulsive disorder (up to 5–15%)
- Personality disorder (5–15%)

Negative symptoms

- Blunted affect
- Emotional withdrawal
- Poor rapport
- Passive/apathetic social withdrawal
- Difficulty in abstract thinking
- Lack of spontaneity and flow of conversation
- Stereotyped thinking

Comorbid symptoms
(below diagnostic threshold)

- Depressive symptoms (40–60%)
- Manic symptoms (10–30%)
- Personality traits (20–50%)
- Social anxiety (10–20%)
- Obsessive–compulsive symptoms (20–30%)

Figure 4.3 Symptoms, comorbid psychiatric symptoms and disorders, and resulting psychosocial dysfunctions in patients with schizophrenia. Adapted from Lambert et al [23].

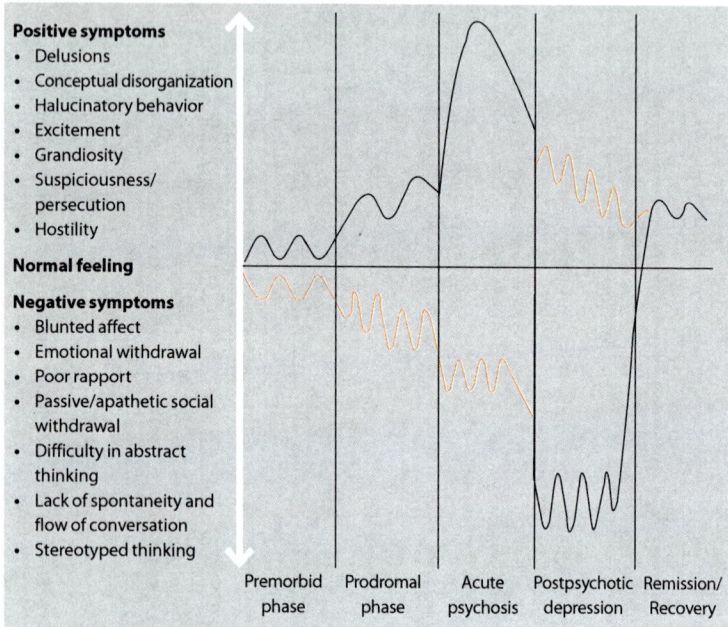

Model of positive and negative symptoms and value of symptoms during the course of schizophrenia

Positive symptoms
- Delusions
- Conceptual disorganization
- Halucinatory behavior
- Excitement
- Grandiosity
- Suspiciousness/ persecution
- Hostility

Normal feeling

Negative symptoms
- Blunted affect
- Emotional withdrawal
- Poor rapport
- Passive/apathetic social withdrawal
- Difficulty in abstract thinking
- Lack of spontaneity and flow of conversation
- Stereotyped thinking

| Premorbid phase | Prodromal phase | Acute psychosis | Postpsychotic depression | Remission/ Recovery |

Figure 4.4 Model of positive and negative symptoms and value of symptoms during the course of schizophrenia. Adapted from Lambert et al [23].

There is some controversy over whether the disorganized symptoms are a separate set of symptoms of schizophrenia or whether, as they are seen in other presentations (eg, manic phase of bipolar disorder), they should not be considered diagnostic of schizophrenia on their own.

At present, schizophrenia is mainly defined by the presence of positive symptoms. However, there are those who see it as more of a cognitive disorder, with the presence of neurocognitive deficits being a marked feature of the presentation in many people with schizophrenia (see Figure 4.3).

Psychosocial assessment

In line with the complexity of the disorder, the psychosocial assessment in schizophrenia includes a mental state examination, a risk assessment, an assessment of the personal and psychiatric history and comorbid psychiatric disorders, and an assessment of possible social problems (Figure 4.5).

Overview of major aspects of the psychosocial assessment in schizophrenia

Assessment	Content
Mental State Examination	• Positive symptoms (eg, hallucinations, systematized delusions) • Negative symptoms (eg, primary deficit syndrome, secondary negative symptoms) • Disorganization, thought disorder • Manic or depressive syndromes, anxiety • Cognitive dysfunctions • Insight
Risk assessment	• Suicidal risk (eg, actual thoughts or plans, past suicide attempts, depression, delusion-related anxiety, substance use, command hallucinations, tragic loss) • Violent/aggressive behavior (eg, previous violent behavior, agitation, disorganization, suspiciousness/delusions, dysphoric and/or manic symptoms, antisocial personality, catatonic excitement, drug intoxication) • Risk of victimization by others (eg, disorganization, manic–psychotic mental state) • Risk of treatment nonadherence (eg, insufficient therapeutic alliance, persistent comorbid substance abuse disorder, lack of insight, negative attitude toward medication, negative subjective wellbeing under antipsychotics, lack of social support) • Risk of service disengagement and unauthorized absconding from hospital (eg, young age, male, persistent substance use disorder, antisocial personality, lack of insight)
Personal and psychiatric history	• Biography (eg, developmental milestones, school/work status and functioning, peer relationships) • Psychiatric history of family (eg, psychiatric disorders in relatives, expressed emotion, genetic risk) • Pregnancy and obstetric complications (eg, intrauterine infection, hypoxia, premature birth) • Early developmental events (eg, delayed speaking and walking) • Functional problems during early childhood (eg, in kindergarten or elementary school) • Premorbid functioning • Trauma in early childhood or youth and other psychosocial stressors • Prodromal symptoms (including Brief Limited Intermittant Psychotic Symptoms [BLIPS], Attenuated Positive Symptoms [APS], reduced functioning level in the last 12 months, duration of prodrome, time point of ongoing positive symptom manifestation) • Duration of untreated psychosis (including symptoms and symptomatic development) • Forensic history • Pathways to care • Psychodynamic context

Figure 4.5 Overview of major aspects of the psychosocial assessment in schizophrenia (continues overleaf).

Overview of major aspects of the psychosocial assessment in schizophrenia (continued)

Assessment	Content
Comorbid psychiatric disorders	• Comorbid psychiatric disorder (premorbid, during prodrome, during untreated psychosis, and at initial presentation)
	• Substance abuse disorder (eg, type, abuse or dependency, onset, actual use, reasons for use, previous treatment, previous drug-induced psychosis, motivation to change)
	• Major depression (eg, onset, course, previous treatment, actual severity)
	• Anxiety disorder (eg, onset, course, previous treatment, severity; especially social phobia and post-traumatic stress disorder)
	• Obsessive–compulsive disorder (eg, onset, course, previous treatment, severity)
	• Personality disorder/traits (eg, onset, course, previous treatment, severity; especially antisocial and avoidant personality disorder)
	• Learning disability
	• Attention-deficit/hyperactivity disorder

Figure 4.5 Overview of major aspects of the psychosocial assessment in schizophrenia (continued).

Neuromedical assessment

A full neuromedical examination should be undertaken. This examination is important for detection of comorbidities and risk factors for future somatic diseases, especially cardiovascular disease, including obesity, smoking, hypertension, dyslipidemia, and type 2 diabetes. Furthermore, the medical assessment gives information on the potential existence of an organic cause of psychosis and whether there are risk factors for incomplete remission or treatment resistance (eg, wide ventricles on magnetic resonance tomography). It also establishes a baseline against which possible future side effects and complications of pharmacologic treatment can be measured.

Neuropsychologic assessment

Approximately 75% of patients with schizophrenia display cognitive dysfunctions in a wide variety of domains [24] (see Chapter 2, page 19). Cognitive assessment is important because empirical evidence has shown that cognitive deficits are determinants of functional outcome. Furthermore, they are linked to other clinical variables such as insight or the ability to take medication as prescribed. Moreover, undisturbed cognitive abilities are important for patients to benefit successfully from psychotherapeutic interventions. The assessment should be undertaken when the patient is not acutely psychotic and has been stabilized. A repeated assessment is recommended about 6 months after the first neuropsychologic test.

Assessment of psychotic and comorbid psychiatric disorders

The diagnostic categorization of schizophrenia is hampered by several factors (eg, diagnostic instability, a large range of differential diagnoses [Figure 4.6], and a high rate of comorbid psychiatric disorders).

Formulation of the diagnosis of schizophrenia includes assessment of specific symptoms and their duration, as well as exclusion of other psychotic disorders. The most important differential diagnoses are schizoaffective or bipolar disorder type I, delusional disorder, psychosis (not otherwise specified), borderline personality disorder, and major depression with psychotic features. The differential diagnosis of a schizophreniform disorder differs in duration of psychotic symptoms but not in type of symptoms. Psychotic episodes shorter than 1 month (the *International Classification of Diseases, 10th Revision* [ICD-10]) or 6 months (*Diagnostic and Statistical Manual of Mental Disorders, 4th Edition* [DSM-IV]) are diagnosed as schizophreniform disorder [25,26]. Other types of psychosis must be considered as well. However, since the introduction of the 6-month duration criterion with DSM-III, schizophrenia is reported to be the most stable diagnosis (about 90%) over a period of 6 months to 40 years.

The diagnosis should be made using modern operationalized systems, such as the ICD-10 or DSM-IV. Both systems require exactly defined criteria to be met for the diagnosis of schizophrenia. The diagnosis of schizophrenia can be made only if specifically defined symptoms have been present for a predefined period and other etiologies have been excluded. As schizophrenia is a heterogeneous disorder, generally, subtypes are differentiated. These are not disorders themselves, but rather descriptions of predominant psychopathology. The subtypes of schizophrenia differ from each other according to the predominant psychopathology

Differential diagnosis of schizophrenia according to ICD-10 or DSM-IV

ICD-10/DSM-IV	Differential diagnosis
F0/290, 293, 294 Organic, including symptomatic mental disorders	• Encephalitis (eg, herpes encephalitis, AIDS encephalitis, Creutzfeldt–Jakob, neurosyphilis) • Traumatic cerebral injury • Cerebral tumors • Epilepsy • Hormonal disorders (eg, Cushing's syndrome, hyperthyroidism) • Neurodegenerative disorders (such as dementia, Friedreich's ataxia, Huntington's disease, Parkinson's disease) • Endocrine disorders (such as acute intermittent porphyria, Wilson's disease, uremia, vitamin B_{12} insufficiency, zinc insufficiency) • Rheumatic disorders (eg, lupus erythematosus) • Multiple sclerosis • Others (narcolepsy, pregnancy, heart disorders, endocrinopathies, postoperative states)
F1/291–305 Mental and behavioral disorders due to psychotropic substances	• Drug-induced psychotic disorder • Intoxication • Withdrawal syndrome with or without delirium
F2/293–298 Schizophrenia spectrum disorders	• Brief psychotic episode • Schizophreniform disorder (ICD-10: ≤1 month; DSM-IV: ≤6 months) • Schizoaffective disorder (manic, mixed, and depressive type) • Delusional disorder • Drug-induced psychotic disorder (for subtype see F1 in ICD-10 or pages 291–305 in DSM-IV-TR) • Psychotic disorder (not otherwise specified) • Schizotypal disorder • Acute transient delusional disorder • Induced delusional disorder
F3/293–296 Affective disorders	• Bipolar affective disorder (manic, mixed, and depressive type) • Severe depressive episode with psychotic symptoms • Recurrent depressive disorder, presently severe depressive episode, with psychotic symptoms
F4/300.01–309.9 Neurotic, stress, and somatioform disorders	• Dissociative stupor • Depersonalization and derealization syndrome
F6/301.0–301.9 Personality and behavioral disorders	• Paranoid personality disorder • Schizoid personality disorder • Emotionally unstable personality disorder (borderline type) • Artificial disorders
F8 Developmental disorders	• Asperger's syndrome • Autistic spectrum disorders

Figure 4.6 Differential diagnosis of schizophrenia according to ICD-10 or DSM-IV. Adapted from the World Health Organization [25] and the American Psychiatric Association [26].

and certain time criteria. The most common subtype is the paranoid subtype, but a change of subtypes in the course of illness as a result of changing psychopathology is often possible.

If the type of psychotic disorder or the existence and type of comorbid disorders remain unclear, both can be assessed with structured diagnostic interviews when the patient is stabilized (eg, Structured Clinical Interview for DSM-IV). For first-episode psychosis patients such an interview should be repeated 12 months after the initial episode. This recommendation is based on studies that show that up to 40% of initial diagnoses need to be changed within 12 months. With the exception of substance abuse disorders, the diagnostic evaluation of comorbid psychiatric disorders is often difficult (see Figure 4.5). As untreated comorbid psychiatric disorders can worsen the course of schizophrenia, they should be consequently assessed and treated.

Useful assessment scales

At-risk criteria
- Schizophrenia Proneness Instrument, Adult version (SPI-A) or Child and Youth version (SPI-CY)
- Structured Interview for Psychosis-Risk Syndromes (SIPS)
- Comprehensive Assessment of At-Risk Mental States (CAARMS)

Positive, negative, and general symptoms
- Positive and Negative Syndrome Scale (PANSS)
- Brief Psychiatric Rating Scale (BPRS)
- Scale for Assessment of Positive Symptoms (SAPS)
- Scale for Assessment of Negative Symptoms (SANS)

Severity of illness
- Clinical Global Impression Scale (CGI)
- Clinical Global Impression Scale – Schizophrenia version (CGI-Sch)

Level of functioning
- Global Assessment of Functioning Scale (GAF)
- Scale of Occupational and Functional Assessment (SOFAS)
- Role Functioning Scale (RFS)

Specific comorbid symptoms
- Calgary Depression Symptoms Scale (CDSS)
- Beck Depression Inventory (BDI)

Beck Hopelessness Scale (BHS)

Quality of life
- Quality of Life Enjoyment and Satisfaction Questionnaire (Q-LES-Q-18)
- MOS 36-Item Short-Form Health Survey (SF-36)
- Drug Attitude Inventory (DAI)

Subjective wellbeing under neuroleptic treatment
- Subjective Wellbeing under Neuroleptic Treatment (SWN-K), short form

Service engagement, satisfaction with care, medication adherence
- Service Engagement Scale (SES)
- Client Satisfaction Questionnaire (CSQ-8)
- Satisfaction with Antipsychotic Medication scale (SWAM)
- Medication Adherence Rating Scale (MARS)

Other resources

Psychiatric associations and major national websites
- UK and Ireland
  - National Institute for Health and Clinical Excellence (NHS): http://www.nice.org.uk/Docref.asp?d=62331
  - PsychNet-UK: www.psychnet-uk.com
  - Royal College of Physicians : www.rcpsych.ac.uk
  - Rethink Mental Illness: www.rethink.org
- USA and Canada
  - American Psychiatric Association (APA): www.psych.org
  - National Institute of Mental Health: www.nimh.nih.gov
  - Schizophrenia Society of Canada: www.schizophrenia.ca
  - Canadian Psychiatric Association (CPA): www.cpa-apc.org
  - Canadian Mental Health Association: www.cmha.ca

- Germany
  - German Association of Psychiatry, Psychotherapy, and Neurology (DGPPN): www.dgppn.de
  - Research Network on Schizophrenia: www.kompetenznetz-schizophrenie.de
  - Currently Psychiatry: www.psychiatrie-aktuell.de/homes/schizophrenia.jhtml
  - Schizophrenia Network: www.psychose-netz.de/news.php
- Australia
  - Royal Australian and New Zealand College of Psychiatrists: www.ranzcp.org
  - Orygen Youth Health: www.orygen.org.au
- International
  - Schizophrenia International Research Society: www.schizophreniaresearchsociety.org

Information for patients and relatives

- www.schizophrenia.com
- www.psychosis-bipolar.com
- www.psychose.de (in German)
- www.psihos.ru (in Russian)
- www.psychose.de/tr (in Turkish)
- www.sane.org.uk
- www.mind.org.uk
- www.psychnet-uk.com
- www.rcpsych.ac.uk
- www.schizophrenia-world.org.uk
- www.sane.org
- www.eufami.org
- www.gamian.org

References

1   McGrath J, Saha S, Welham J, El Saadi O, MacCauley C, Chant D. A systematic review of the incidence of schizophrenia: the distribution of rates and the influence of sex, urbanicity, migrant status and methodology. *BMC Med.* 2004;2:13.

2   Saha S, Chant D, Welham J, McGrath J. A systematic review of the prevalence of schizophrenia. *PLoS Med.* 2005;2:e141.

3   Amminger GP, Harris MG, Conus P, et al. Treated incidence of first-episode psychosis in the catchment area of EPPIC between 1997 and 2000. *Acta Psychiatr Scand.* 2006;114:337-345.

4   Messias EL, Chen CY, Eaton WW. Epidemiology of schizophrenia: review of findings and myths. *Psychiatr Clin North Am.* 2007;30:323-338.

5   Remschmidt H, Theisen FM. Schizophrenia and related disorders in children and adolescents. *J Neural Transm Suppl.* 2005;69:121-141.

6   Howard R, Rabins PV, Seeman MV, Jeste DV; The International Late-Onset Schizophrenia Group. Late-onset schizophrenia and very-late-onset schizophrenia-like psychosis: an international consensus. *Am J Psychiatry.* 2000;157:172-178.

7   Harrison P, Geddes J,SharpeM. *Lecture Notes: Psychiatry.* 10th edn. Chichester, UK: Wiley-Blackwell; 2010.

8   Lambert M. *Taschenatlas der Pharmakotherapie psychotischer Störungen.* Stuttgart, Germany: Thieme-Verlag, 2009.

9   Hallmayer J. The epidemiology of the genetic liability for schizophrenia. *Aust N Z J Psychiatry.* 2000;34(suppl):S47-S55.

10 McGue M, Gottesman II, Rao DC. Resolving genetic models for the transmission of schizophrenia. *Genet Epidemiol.* 1985;2:99-110.

11 Kety SS, Wender PH, Jacobsen B, et al. Mental illness in the biological and adoptive relatives of schizophrenic adoptees: replication of the Copenhagen Study in the rest of Denmark. *Arch Gen Psychiatry.* 1994;51:442-455.

12 Mamah D, Barch DM. Diagnosis and classification of the schizophrenia spectrum disorders. In: Ritsner MS, ed. *Handbook of Schizophrenia Spectrum Disorders. Volume I: Conceptual Issues and Neurobiological Advances.* Dordrecht, The Netherlands: Springer Science + Business Media; 2011:45-84.

13 Larsen TK, Friis S, Haahr U, et al. Early detection and intervention in first-episode schizophrenia: a critical review. *Acta Psychiatr Scand.* 2001;103:323-334.

14 American Psychiatric Association. Practice Guideline for the Treatment of Patients with Schizophrenia, 2nd compendium. Arlington, VA: APA, 2004.

15 Häfner H, Maurer K, Löffler W, Riecher-Rössler A. The influence of age and sex on the onset and early course of schizophrenia. *Br J Psychiatry.* 1993;162:80-86.

16 Currier GW, Allen MH. Emergency psychiatry: physical and chemical restraint in the psychiatric emergency service. *Psychiatr Serv.* 2000;51:717-719.

17 Regier DA, Farmer ME, Rae DS, Locke BZ, Keith SJ, Judd LL, Goodwin FK. Comorbidity of mental disorders with alcohol and other drug abuse. Results from the Epidemiologic Catchment Area (ECA) Study. *JAMA.* 1990;264:2511-2518.

18 Caldwell CB, Gottesman II. Schizophrenics kill themselves, too: a review of risk factors for suicide. *Schizophr Bull.* 1990;16:571-589.

19 Shepherd M, Watt D, Falloon I, Smeeton N. The natural history of schizophrenia: a five-year follow-up study of outcome and prediction in a representative sample of schizophrenics. *Psychol Med Monogr Suppl.* 1989;15:1-46.

20 Bleuler M. A 23-year longitudinal study of 208 schizophrenics and impressions in regard to the nature of schizophrenia. In: Rosenthal D, Kety S, eds. *The Transmission Of Schizophrenia.* New York, NY: Pergamon Press; 1968:3-12.

21 Winokur G, Pfohl B, Tsuang, M. A 40-year follow-up of hebephrenic-catatonic schizophrenia. In Miller NE, Cohen GD, eds. *Schizophrenia and Aging.* New York, NY: Guilford Press; 1987.

22 Steinmeyer EM, Marneros A, Deister A, Rohde A, Jünemann H. Long-term outcome of schizoaffective and schizophrenic disorders: a comparative study. II. Causal-analytical investigations. *Eur Arch Psychiatry Neurol Sci.* 1989;238:126-34.

23 Lambert M, Bäuml J. Schlag auf, sieh nach: Psychosen - ein Handbuch für Betreuer und medizinisches Personal. Saarbrücken, Germany: VDM Verlag; 2009.

24 O'Carroll R. Cognitive impairment in schizophrenia. Adv Psych Treat. 2000;6:161-168.

25 World Health Organization. The ICD-10 Classification of Mental and Behavioural Disorders, Clinical Descriptions and Diagnostic Guidelines. Geneva, Switzerland: World Health Organization; 1992.

26 American Psychiatric Association. Diagnostic and Statistical Manual of Mental Disorders (Text Revision). 4th edn. Washington, DC: American Psychiatric Press; 1994.

Further reading

The following list comprises key literature on schizophrenia. To facilitate easy access to the most important articles and reviews, the list is sorted alphabetically according to different topics.

Behavioral emergencies

Allen MH, Currier GW, Hughes DH, et al. Expert consensus panel for behavioral emergencies. The Expert Consensus Guideline Series. Treatment of behavioral emergencies. *Postgrad Med*. 2001;1-88.

Allen MH, Currier GW, Carpenter D, et al. Treatment of behavioral emergencies. *J Psychiatr Pract*. 2005;11:5-108.

Hankin CS, Bronstone A, Koran LM. Agitation in the inpatient psychiatric setting: a review of clinical presentation, burden, and treatment. *J Psychiatr Pract*. 2011;17:170-185.

Huband N, Ferriter M, Nathan R, Jones H. Antiepileptics for aggression and associated impulsivity. *Cochrane Database Syst Rev*. 2010;(2):CD003499.

Lambert M, Huber CG, Naber D, et al. Treatment of severe agitation with olanzapine in an unselected cohort of 166 patients with schizophrenia, schizoaffective or bipolar I disorder. *Pharmacopsychiatry*. 2008;41:182-189.

Marco CA, Vaughan J. Emergency management of agitation in schizophrenia. *Am J Emerg Med*. 2005;23:767-776.

Montoya A, Valladares A, Lizán L, San L, Escobar R, Paz S. Validation of the excited component of the Positive and Negative Syndrome Scale (PANSS-EC) in a naturalistic sample of 278 patients with acute psychosis and agitation in a psychiatric emergency room. *Health Qual Life Outcomes*. 2011;9:18.

Thomas P, Alptekin K, Gheorghe M, Mauri M, Olivares JM, Riedel M. Management of patients presenting with acute psychotic episodes of schizophrenia. *CNS Drugs*. 2009;23:193-212.

Topiwala A, Fazel S. The pharmacological management of violence in schizophrenia: a structured review. *Expert Rev Neurother*. 2011;11:53-63.

Volavka J, Citrome L. Pathways to aggression in schizophrenia affect results of treatment. *Schizophr Bull*. 2011;37:921-929.

Childhood trauma

Bebbington PE, Bhugra D, Brugha T, et al. Psychosis, victimisation and childhood disadvantage: evidence from the second British National Survey of Psychiatric Morbidity. *Br J Psychiatry*. 2004;185:220-226.

Conus P, Cotton S, Schimmelmann BG, et al. Pretreatment and outcome correlates of past sexual and physical trauma in 118 bipolar I disorder patients with a first episode of psychotic mania. *Bipolar Disorder*. 2010;12:244-252.

Morgan C, Fisher H. Environment and schizophrenia: environmental factors in schizophrenia: childhood trauma–a critical review. *Schizophr Bull*. 2007;33:3-10.

M. Lambert and D. Naber, *Current Schizophrenia*,
DOI: 10.1007/978-1-908517-68-5,
© Springer Healthcare, a part of Springer Science+Business Media 2012

Mueser KT, Rosenberg SD, Xie H, et al. A randomized controlled trial of cognitive-behavioral treatment for posttraumatic stress disorder in severe mental illness. *J Consult Clin Psychol.* 2008;76:259-271.

Read J, van Os J, Morrison AP, Ross CA. Childhood trauma, psychosis and schizophrenia: A literature review with theoretical and clinical implications. *Acta Psychiatr Scand.* 2005;112:330-350.

Read J. Breaking the silence: learning why, when and how to ask about trauma, and how to respond to disclosures. In: Larkin W, Morrison A, eds. *Trauma and Psychosis.* London, UK: Brunner-Routledge; 2006:195-221.

Schäfer I, Ross CA, Read J. Childhood trauma. In: Moskowitz A, Schäfer I, Dorahy M, eds. *Psychosis, Trauma, and Dissociation: Emerging Perspectives on Severe Psychopathology.* London: John Wiley & Sons; 2008:137-150.

Childhood-onset schizophrenia

Gentile S. Clinical usefulness of second-generation antipsychotics in treating children and adolescents diagnosed with bipolar or schizophrenic disorders. *Paediatr Drugs.* 2011;13:291-302.

Gogtay N, Vyas NS, Testa R, Wood SJ, Pantelis C. Age of onset of schizophrenia: perspectives from structural neuroimaging studies. *Schizophr Bull.* 2011;37 504-513.

Kennedy E, Kumar A, Datta SS. Antipsychotic medication for childhood-onset schizophrenia. *Cochrane Database Syst Rev.* 2007;(3):CD004027.

Madaan V, Dvir Y, Wilson DR. Child and adolescent schizophrenia: pharmacological approaches. *Expert Opin Pharmacother.* 2008;9:2053-2068.

Masi G, Liboni F. Management of schizophrenia in children and adolescents: focus on pharmacotherapy. *Drugs.* 2011;71:179-208.

Mattai AK, Hill JL, Lenroot RK. Treatment of early-onset schizophrenia. *Curr Opin Psychiatry.* 2010;23:304-310.

Rapoport JL, Gogtay N. Childhood onset schizophrenia: support for a progressive neurodevelopmental disorder. *Int J Dev Neurosci.* 2011;29:251-258.

Classifications of psychotic disorders

American Psychiatric Association. *Diagnostic and Statistical Manual of Mental Disorders (Text Revision).* 4th edn. Washington, DC: American Psychiatric Press; 1994.

World Health Organization. *The ICD-10 Classification of Mental and Behavioural Disorders, Clinical Descriptions and Diagnostic Guidelines.* Geneva, Switzerland: World Health Organization; 1992.

Duration of antipsychotic treatment

Bosveld-van Haandel LJ, Slooff CJ, van den Bosch RJ. Reasoning about the optimal duration of prophylactic antipsychotic medication in schizophrenia: evidence and arguments. *Acta Psychiatr Scand.* 2001;103:335-346.

Gitlin M, Nuechterlein K, Subotnik KL, et al. Clinical outcome following neuroleptic discontinuation in patients with remitted recent-onset schizophrenia. *Am J Psychiatry.* 2001;158:1835-1842.

Early intervention and prodromal schizophrenia

Amminger GP, Schäfer MR, Papageorgiou K, et al. Long-chain omega-3 fatty acids for indicated prevention of psychotic disorders: a randomized, placebo-controlled trial. *Arch Gen Psychiatry.* 2010;67:146-154.

Bechdolf A, Wagner M, Ruhrmann S, et al. Preventing progression to first-episode psychosis in early initial prodromal states. *Br J Psychiatry.* 2012;200:22-29.

Bodatsch M, Ruhrmann S, Wagner M, et al. Prediction of psychosis by mismatch negativity. *Biol Psychiatry.* 2011;69:959-966.

Correll CU, Hauser M, Auther AM, Cornblatt BA. Research in people with psychosis risk syndrome: a review of the current evidence and future directions. *J Child Psychol Psychiatry.* 2010;51:390-431.

Francey SM, Nelson B, Thompson A, et al. Who needs antipsychotic medication in the earliest stages of psychosis? A reconsideration of benefits, risks, neurobiology and ethics in the era of early intervention. *Schizophr Res.* 2010;119:1-10.

French P, Morrisson AP. *Early Detection and Cognitive Therapy for People at High Risk of Developing Psychosis. A Treatment Approach.* Chichester, UK: Wiley; 2004.

Howes OD, Montgomery AJ, Asselin MC, et al. Elevated striatal dopamine function linked to prodromal signs of schizophrenia. *Arch Gen Psychiatry.* 2009;66:13-20.

Klosterkotter J, Hellmich M, Steinmeyer EM, Schultze-Lutter F. Diagnosing schizophrenia in the initial prodromal phase. *Arch Gen Psychiatry.* 2001;58:158-164.

Koch E, Schultze-Lutter F, Schimmelmann BG, Resch F. On the importance and detection of prodromal symptoms from the perspective of child and adolescent psychiatry. *Clin Neuropsych.* 2010;7:38-48.

Koutsouleris N, Meisenzahl EM, Davatzikos C, et al. Use of neuroanatomical pattern classification to identify subjects in at-risk mental states of psychosis and predict disease transition. *Arch Gen Psychiatry.* 2009;66:700-712.

Larson MK, Walker EF, Compton MT. Early signs, diagnosis and therapeutics of the prodromal phase of schizophrenia and related psychotic disorders. *Expert Rev Neurother.* 2010;10:1347-1359.

Marshall M, Rathbone J. Early intervention for psychosis. *Cochrane Database Syst Rev.* 2011;(6):CD004718.

McGlashan TH, Zipursky RB, Perkins D, et al. Randomized, double-blind trial of olanzapine versus placebo in patients prodromally symptomatic for psychosis. *Am J Psychiat.* 2006;163:790-799.

McGorry PD, Nelson B, Amminger GP, et al. Intervention in individuals at ultra high risk of psychosis: a review and future directions. *J Clin Psychiatry.* 2009;70:1206-1212.

McGorry PD, Yung AR, Phillips LJ, et al. Randomized controlled trial of interventions designed to reduce the risk of progression to first-episode psychosis in a clinical sample with subthreshold symptoms. *Arch Gen Psychiat.* 2002;59:921-928.

Mees L, Zdanowicz N, Reynaert C, Jacques D. Adolescents and young adults at ultrahigh risk of psychosis: detection, prediction and treatment. A review of current knowledge. *Psychiatr Danub.* 2011;23(suppl 1):118-122. Morrison AP, French P, Parker S, et al. Three-year follow-up of a randomized controlled trial of cognitive therapy for the prevention of psychosis in people at ultrahigh risk. *Schizophr Bull.* 2007;33:682-687.

O'Brien MP, Zinberg JL, Bearden CE, et al. Psychoeducational multi-family group treatment with adolescents at high risk for developing psychosis. *Early Interv Psychiatry.* 2007;1:325-332.

O'Brien MP, Zinberg JL, Ho L, et al. Family problem solving interactions and 6-month symptomatic and functional outcomes in youth at ultra-high risk for psychosis and with recent onset psychotic symptoms: a longitudinal study. *Schizophr Res.* 2009;107:198-205.

Phillips LJ, McGorry PD, Yuen HP, et al. Medium term follow-up of a randomized controlled trial of interventions for young people at ultra high risk of psychosis. *Schizophr Res.* 2007;96:25-33.

Preti A, Cella M. Randomized-controlled trials in people at ultra high risk of psychosis: a review of treatment effectiveness. *Schizophr Res.* 2010;123:30-36.

Pukrop R, Klosterkotter J. Neurocognitive indicators of clinical high-risk states for psychosis: a critical review of the evidence. *Neurotox Res.* 2010;18:272-286.

Ruhrmann S, Bechdolf A, Kuhn KU, et al. Acute effects of treatment for prodromal symptoms for people putatively in a late initial prodromal state of psychosis. *Br J Psychiatry.* 2007;51:s88-s95.

Ruhrmann S, Paruch J, Bechdolf A, et al. Reduced subjective quality of life in persons at risk for psychosis. *Acta Psychiatrica Scandinavica.* 2008;117(5): 357-368.

Ruhrmann S, Schultze-Lutter F, Salokangas RK, et al. Prediction of Psychosis in Adolescents and Young Adults – Results from a Prospective European Multicenter Study (EPOS). *Arch Gen Psychiatry.* 2010;67:241-251.

Ruhrmann S, Schultze-Lutter F, Schimmelmann B, Klosterkotter J. Prevention and early intervention in at-risk states for developing psychosis. In: Ritsner M, ed. *Textbook of Schizophrenia Spectrum Disorders*, Volume III. Dordrecht, the Netherlands: Springer Science + Business Media; 2011:81-92.

Ruhrmann S, Schultze-Lutter F, Klosterkötter J. Early detection and intervention in the initial prodromal phase of schizophrenia. *Pharmacopsychiatry.* 2003;36(suppl 3):162-167.

Ruhrmann S, Schultze-Lutter F, Klosterkotter J. Sub-threshold states of psychosis – a challenge to diagnosis and treatment. *Clin Neuropsych.* 2010;7:72-87.

Schultze-Lutter F, Klosterkotter J, Picker H, Steinmeyer EM, Ruhrmann S. Predicting first-episode psychosis by basic symptom criteria. *Clin Neuropsych.* 2007;4:11-22.

Schultze-Lutter F, Michel C, Ruhrmann S, Klosterkotter J, Schimmelmann B. Prediction and early detection of first-episode psychosis. In: Ritsner M, ed. *Textbook of Schizophrenia Spectrum Disorders*, Volume II. Dordrecht, the Netherlands: Springer Science + Business Media; 2007:207-268.

Simon AE, Dvorsky DN, Boesch J, et al. Defining subjects at risk for psychosis: A comparison of two approaches. *Schizophr Res.* 2006;81:83-90.

Smieskova R, Fusar-Poli P, Allen P, et al. Neuroimaging predictors of transition to psychosis - a systematic review and meta-analysis. *Neurosci Biobehav Rev.* 2010;34:1207-1222.

Wölwer W, Brinkmeyer J, Stroth S, et al. Neurophysiological correlates of impaired facial affect recognition in individuals at risk for schizophrenia. Schizophr Bull. 2011. [Ebup ahead of print]Yung AR, McGorry PD, McFarlane CA, Jackson HJ, Patton GC, Rakkar A. Monitoring and care of young people at incipient risk of psychosis. *Schizophrenia Bull.* 1996;22:283-303.

Yung AR, Nelson B. Young people at ultra high risk for psychosis: a research update. *Early Interv Psychiatry.* 2011;5(suppl 1):52-57.

Electroconvulsive therapy

Read J, Bentall R. The effectiveness of electroconvulsive therapy: a literature review. *Epidemiol Psichiatr Soc.* 2010;19:333-347.

Tharyan P, Adams CE. Electroconvulsive therapy for schizophrenia. *Cochrane Database Syst Rev.* 2005;2:CD000076.

Epidemiology and etiology

Brown AS. The environment and susceptibility to schizophrenia. *Prog Neurobiol.* 2011;93:23-58.

Cannon M, Jones PB, Murray RM. Obstetric complications and schizophrenia: historical and meta-analytic review. *Am J Psychiatry.* 2002;159:1080-1092.

Goldner EM, Hsu L, Waraich P, Somers JM. Prevalence and incidence studies of schizophrenic disorders: a systematic review of the literature. *Can J Psychiatry.* 2002;47:833-843.

Haraldsson HM, Ettinger U, Sigurdsson E. Developments in schizophrenia genetics: from linkage to microchips, deletions and duplications. *Nord J Psychiatry.* 2011;65:82-88.

Malhi GS, Green M, Fagiolini A, Peselow ED, Kumari V. Schizoaffective disorder: diagnostic issues and future recommendations. *Bipolar Disord.* 2008;10:215-230.

Meyer-Lindenberg A. Imaging genetics of schizophrenia. *Dialogues Clin Neurosci.* 2010;12:449-456.

Pickard B. Progress in defining the biological causes of schizophrenia. *Expert Rev Mol Med.* 2011;13:e25.

Schmitt A, Hasan A, Gruber O, Falkai P. Schizophrenia as a disorder of disconnectivity. *Eur Arch Psychiatry Clin Neurosci.* 2011;261(suppl 2):S150-S154.

Tandon R, Keshavan MS, Nasrallah HA. Schizophrenia, "just the facts" what we know in 2008. 2. Epidemiology and etiology. *Schizophr Res.* 2008;102:1-18.

Thornley B, Adams C. Content and quality of 2000 controlled trials in schizophrenia over 50 years. *BMJ.* 2000;317:1181-1184.

van Haren NE, Bakker SC, Kahn RS. Genes and structural brain imaging in schizophrenia. *Curr Opin Psychiatry.* 2008;21:161-167.

van Winkel R, Stefanis NC, Myin-Germeys I. Psychosocial stress and psychosis. A review of the neurobiological mechanisms and the evidence for gene-stress interaction. *Schizophr Bull.* 2008;34:1095-1105.

First-episode psychosis

Bola JR, Kao DT, Soydan H. Antipsychotic medication for early episode schizophrenia. *Cochrane Database Syst Rev.* 2011;(6):CD006374.

Edwards J, McGorry PD. *Implementing Early Intervention in Psychosis.* London: Martin Dunitz; 2002.

Freudenreich O, Holt DJ, Cather C, Goff DC. The evaluation and management of patients with first-episode schizophrenia: a selective, clinical review of diagnosis, treatment, and prognosis. *Harv Rev Psychiatry.* 2007;15:189-211.

Harrigan SM, McGorry PD, Krstev H. Does treatment delay in first-episode psychosis really matter? *Psychol Med.* 2003;33:97-110.

Howard R, Rabins PV, Seeman MV, Jeste DV. Late-onset schizophrenia and very-late-onset schizophrenia-like psychosis: an international consensus. The International Late-Onset schizophrenia group. *Am J Psychiatry.* 2000;157:172-178.

International First Episode Vocational Recovery (iFEVR) Group. Meaningful lives: supporting young people with psychosis in education, training and employment: an international consensus statement. *Early Interv Psychiatry.* 2010;4:323-326.

Killackey E, Yung AR. Effectiveness of early intervention in psychosis. *Curr Opin Psychiatry.* 2007;20:121-125.

Marshall M, Lewis S, Lockwood A, Drake R, Jones P, Croudace T. Association between duration of untreated psychosis and outcome in cohorts of first-episode patients: a systematic review. *Arch Gen Psychiatry.* 2005;62:975-983.

McGorry PD, Edwards J, Mihalopoulos C, Harrigan SM, Jackson HJ. EPPIC: an evolving system of early detection and optimal management. *Schizophr Bull.* 1996;22:305-322.

Pompili M, Serafini G, Innamorati M, et al. Suicide risk in first episode psychosis: a selective review of the current literature. *Schizophr Res.* 2011;129:1-11.

Robinson D. First-episode schizophrenia. *CNS Spectr.* 2010;15(suppl 6):4-7.

Schimmelmann BG, Huber CG, Lambert M, Cotton S, McGorry PD, Conus P. Impact of duration of untreated psychosis on initial presentation and outcome in an epidemiological first episode psychosis cohort. *J Psychiatr Res.* 2008;42:982-990.

Late-onset schizophrenia

Chan WC, Lam LC, Chen EY. Recent advances in pharmacological treatment of psychosis in late life. *Curr Opin Psychiatry.* 2011;24:455-460.

Marriott RG, Neil W, Waddingham S. Antipsychotic medication for elderly people with schizophrenia. *Cochrane Database Syst Rev.* 2006;(1):CD005580.

New antipsychotics and new antipsychotic formulations

Overview

Chue P, Emsley R. Long-acting formulations of atypical antipsychotics: time to reconsider when to introduce depot antipsychotics. *CNS Drugs*. 2007;21:441-448.

Citrome L. Iloperidone, asenapine, and lurasidone: a brief overview of 3 new second-generation antipsychotics. *Postgrad Med*. 2010;123:153-162.

Correll CU. From receptor pharmacology to improved outcomes: individualising the selection, dosing, and switching of antipsychotics. *Eur Psychiatry*. 2010;25(suppl 2):S12-S21.

Haddad P, Lambert T, Lauriello J. The role of antipsychotic long-acting injections in current practice. In Haddad P, Lambert T, Lauriello J, eds. *Antipsychotic Long-Acting Injections*. Oxford, UK: Oxford University Press; 2011:241-260.

Kane JM, Garcia-Ribera C. Clinical guideline recommendations for antipsychotic long-acting injections. *Br J Psychiatry*. 2009;195:63-67.

Lambert T, Taylor D. Pharmacology of antipsychotic long-acting injections. In Haddad P, Lambert T, Lauriello J, eds. *Antipsychotic Long-Acting Injections*. Oxford, UK: Oxford University Press; 2011:23-46.

Leucht C, Heres S, Kane JM, Kissling W, Davis JM, Leucht S. Oral versus depot antipsychotic drugs for schizophrenia – a critical systematic review and meta-analysis of randomised long-term trials. *Schizophr Res*. 2011;127:83-92.

Asenapine

Citrome L. Asenapine for schizophrenia and bipolar disorder: a review of the efficacy and safety profile for this newly approved sublingually absorbed second-generation antipsychotic. *Int J Clin Pract*. 2009;63:1762-1784.

McIntyre RS. Asenapine: a review of acute and extension phase data in bipolar disorder. *CNS Neurosci Ther*. 2011;17:645-848.

Minassian A, Young JW. Evaluation of the clinical efficacy of asenapine in schizophrenia. *Exp Opin Pharmacother*. 2010;11:2107-2115.

Pompili M, Serafini G, Innamorati M, et al. Unmet treatment needs in schizophrenia patients: is asenapine a potential therapeutic option? *Expert Rev Neurother*. 2011;11:989-1006.

Iloperidone

Arif SA, Mitchell MM. Iloperidone: a new drug for the treatment of schizophrenia. *Am J Health Syst Pharm*. 2011;68:301-308.

Citrome L. Iloperidone: chemistry, pharmacodynamics, pharmacokinetics and metabolism, clinical efficacy, safety and tolerability, regulatory affairs, and an opinion. *Expert Opin Drug Metab Toxicol*. 2010;6:1551-1564.

Crabtree BL, Montgomery J. Iloperidone for the management of adults with schizophrenia. *Clin Ther*. 2011;33:330-345.

Lurasidone

Citrome L. Lurasidone for schizophrenia: a brief review of a new second-generation antipsychotic. *Clin Schizophr Relat Psychoses*. 2011;4:251-257.

Citrome L. Lurasidone for schizophrenia: a review of the efficacy and safety profile for this newly approved second-generation antipsychotic. *Int J Clin Pract*. 2011;65:189-210.

Meltzer HY, Cucchiaro J, Silva R, et al. Lurasidone in the treatment of schizophrenia: a randomized, double-blind, placebo- and olanzapine-controlled study. *Am J Psychiatry*. 2011;168:957-967.

Meyer JM, Loebel AD, Schweizer E. Lurasidone: a new drug in development for schizophrenia. *Expert Opin Investig Drugs*. 2009;18:1715-1726.

Samalin L, Garnier M, Llorca PM. Clinical potential of lurasidone in the management of schizophrenia. *Ther Clin Risk Manag*. 2011;7:239-250.

Olanzapine pamoate

Citrome L. Olanzapine pamoate: a stick in time? A review of the efficacy and safety profile of a new depot formulation of a second-generation antipsychotic. *Int J Clin Pract*. 2009;63:140-150.

Frampton JE. Olanzapine long-acting injection: a review of its use in the treatment of schizophrenia. *Drugs*. 2010;70:2289-2313.

Naber D. Olanzapine pamoate for the treatment of schizophrenia. *Expert Opin Pharmacother*. 2011;12:627-633.

Paliperidone ER

Birnbaum M, Sharif Z. Medication adherence in schizophrenia: patient perspectives and the clinical utility of paliperidone ER. *Patient Prefer Adherence*. 2008;2:233-240.

Canuso CM, Battisti WP. Paliperidone extended-release: a review of efficacy and tolerability in schizophrenia, schizoaffective disorder and bipolar mania. *Expert Opin Pharmacother*. 2010;11:2557-2567.

Gahr M, Kölle MA, Schönfeldt-Lecuona C, Lepping P, Freudenmann RW. Paliperidone extended-release: does it have a place in antipsychotic therapy? *Drug Des Devel Ther*. 2011;5;125-146.

Paliperidone palmitate

Citrome L. Paliperidone palmitate – review of the efficacy, safety and cost of a new second-generation depot antipsychotic medication. *Int J Clin Pract*. 2010;64:216-239.

Gaebel W, Schreiner A, Bergmans P, et al. Relapse prevention in schizophrenia and schizoaffective disorder with risperidone long-acting injectable vs quetiapine: results of a long-term, open-label, randomized clinical trial. *Neuropsychopharmacology*. 2010;35:2367-2377.

Gopal S, Gassmann-Mayer C, Palumbo J, Samtani MN, Shiwach R, Alphs L. Practical guidance for dosing and switching paliperidone palmitate treatment in patients with schizophrenia. *Curr Med Res Opin*. 2010;26:377-387.

Hough D, Gopal S, Vijapurkar U, Lim P, Morozova M, Eerdekens M. Paliperidone palmitate maintenance treatment in delaying the time-to-relapse in patients with schizophrenia: a randomized, double-blind, placebo-controlled study. *Schizophr Res*. 2011;116:107-117.

Hough D, Lindenmayer JP, Gopal S, et al. Safety and tolerability of deltoid and gluteal injections of paliperidone palmitate in schizophrenia. *Prog Neuropsychopharmacol Biol Psychiatry*. 2009;33:1022-1031.

Hoy SM, Scott LJ, Keating GM. Intramuscular paliperidone palmitate. *CNS Drugs*. 2010;24:227-244.

Kramer M, Litman R, Hough D, et al. Paliperidone palmitate, a potential long-acting treatment for patients with schizophrenia. Results of a randomized, double-blind, placebo-controlled efficacy and safety study. *Int J Neuropsychopharmacology*. 2010;13:635-647.

Nasrallah HA, Gopal S, Gassmann-Mayer C, et al. Controlled, evidence-based trial of paliperidone palmitate, long-acting injectable antipsychotic in schizophrenia. *Neuropsychopharmacology*. 2010;35:2072-2082.

Samtani MN, Gopal S, Gassmann-Mayer C, Alphs L, Palumbo JM. Dosing and switching strategies for paliperidone palmitate: based on population pharmacokinetic modelling and clinical trial data. *CNS Drugs.* 2011;25:829-845.

Neuropsychological dysfunctions

Bilder RM, Goldman RS, Robinson D, et al. Neuropsychology of first-episode schizophrenia: initial characterization and clinical correlates. *Am J Psychiatry.* 2000;157:549-559.

Green MF, Kern RS, Braff DL, Mintz J. Neurocognitive deficits and functional outcome in schizophrenia: are we measuring the "right stuff"? *Schizophr Bull.* 2001;26:119-136.

Lewandowski KE, Cohen BM, Ongur D. Evolution of neuropsychological dysfunction during the course of schizophrenia and bipolar disorder. *Psychol Med.* 2011;41:225-241.

Saykin AJ, Shtasel DL, Gur RE, et al. Neuropsychological deficits in neuroleptic naive patients with first-episode schizophrenia. *Arch Gen Psychiatry.* 1994;51:124-131.

Nonadherence and service disengagement

Nonadherence

Goff DC, Hill M, Freudenreich O. Strategies for improving treatment adherence in schizophrenia and schizoaffective disorder. *J Clin Psychiatry.* 2010; 71(suppl 2):20-26.

Gray R, White J, Schulz M, Abderhalden C. Enhancing medication adherence in people with schizophrenia: an international programme of research. *Int J Ment Health Nurs.* 2010;19:36-44.

Kikkert MJ, Schene AH, Koeter MW, et al. Medication adherence in schizophrenia: exploring patients', carers' and professionals' views. *Schizophr Bull.* 2006;32:786-794.

Lacro JP, Dunn LB, Dolder CR, Leckband SG, Jeste DV. Prevalence of and risk factors for medication nonadherence in patients with schizophrenia: a comprehensive review of recent literature. *J Clin Psychiatry.* 2002;63:892-909.

Lambert M, Conus P, Cotton S, Robinson J, McGorry PD, Schimmelmann BG. Prevalence, predictors, and consequences of long-term refusal of antipsychotic treatment in first-episode psychosis. *J Clin Psychopharmacol.* 2010; 30:565-572.

Leucht S, Heres S. Epidemiology, clinical consequences, and psychosocial treatment of nonadherence in schizophrenia. *J Clin Psychiatry.* 2006;67(suppl 5):3-8.

McIntosh AM, Conlon L, Lawrie SM, Stanfield AC. Compliance therapy for schizophrenia. *Cochrane Database Syst Rev.* 2006;(3):CD003442.

Tay SE. Compliance therapy: an intervention to improve inpatients' attitudes toward treatment. *J Psychosoc Nurs Ment Health Serv.* 2007;45:29-37.

Velligan DI, Weiden PJ, Sajatovic M, et al. The expert consensus guideline series: adherence problems in patients with serious and persistent mental illness. *J Clin Psychiatry.* 2009;70(suppl 4):1-46.

Service disengagement

Conus P, Lambert M, Cotton S, Bonsack C, McGorry PD, Schimmelmann BG. Rate and predictors of service disengagement in an epidemiological first-episode psychosis cohort. *Schizophr Res.* 2010;118:256-263.

Kreyenbuhl J, Nossel IR, Dixon LB. Disengagement from mental health treatment among individuals with schizophrenia and strategies for facilitating connections to care: a review of the literature. *Schizophr Bull.* 2009;35:696-703.

Schimmelmann BG, Conus P, Schacht M, McGorry P, Lambert M. Predictors of service disengagement in first-admitted adolescents with psychosis. *J Am Acad Child Adolesc Psychiatry.* 2006;45:990-999.

Pharmacological treatments

Overview

Barnes TR, Schizophrenia Consensus Group of British Association for Psychopharmacology. Evidence-based guidelines for the pharmacological treatment of schizophrenia: recommendations from the British Association for Psychopharmacology. *J Psychopharmacol.* 2011;25:567-620.

Kane JM, Correll CU. Pharmacologic treatment of schizophrenia. *Dialogues Clin Neurosci.* 2010;12:345-357.

Leucht S, Heres S, Kissling W, Davis JM. Evidence-based pharmacotherapy of schizophrenia. *Int J Neuropsychopharmacol.* 2011;14:269-284.

Antipsychotics

Asenjo Lobos C, Komossa K, Rummel-Kluge C, et al. Clozapine versus other atypical antipsychotics for schizophrenia. *Cochrane Database Syst Rev.* 2010;(11):CD006633.

Citrome L. A systematic review of meta-analyses of the efficacy of oral atypical antipsychotics for the treatment of adult patients with schizophrenia. *Expert Opin Pharmacother.* 2012. In press.

Furtado VA, Srihari V. Atypical antipsychotics for people with both schizophrenia and depression. *Cochrane Database Syst Rev.* 2008;(1):CD005377.

Kapur S, Arenovich T, Agid O, Zipursky R, Lindborg S, Jones B. Evidence for onset of antipsychotic effects within the first 24 hours of treatment. *Am J Psychiatry.* 2005;162:939-946.

Lieberman JA, Stroup TS, McEvoy JP, et al. Clinical Antipsychotic Trials of Intervention Effectiveness (CATIE) Investigators. Effectiveness of antipsychotic drugs in patients with chronic schizophrenia. *N Engl J Med.* 2005;353:1209-1223.

McEvoy JP, Hogarty GE, Steingard S. Optimal dose of neuroleptic in acute schizophrenia. A controlled study of the neuroleptic threshold and higher haloperidol dose. *Arch Gen Psychiatry.* 1991;48:739-45.

Potkin SG, Bera R, Gulasekaram B, et al. Plasma clozapine concentrations predict clinical response in treatment-resistant schizophrenia. *J Clin Psychiatry.* 1994;55:133-136.

Spina E, Avenoso A, Facciolà G, et al. Relationship between plasma concentrations of clozapine and norclozapine and therapeutic response in patients with schizophrenia resistant to conventional neuroleptics. *Psychopharmacology.* 2000;148:83-89.

Other medications

Gibson RC, Walcott G. Benzodiazepines for catatonia in people with schizophrenia and other serious mental illnesses. *Cochrane Database Syst Rev.* 2008;(4):CD006570.

Leucht S, Kissling W, McGrath J, White P. Carbamazepine for schizophrenia. *Cochrane Database Syst Rev.* 2007;(3):CD001258.

Leucht S, Kissling W, McGrath J, White P. Lithium for schizophrenia. *Cochrane Database Syst Rev.* 2007;(3):CD003834.

Premkumar TS, Pick J. Lamotrigine for schizophrenia. *Cochrane Database Syst Rev.* 2006;4:CD005962.

Rummel C, Kissling W, Leucht S. Antidepressants for the negative symptoms of schizophrenia. *Cochrane Database Syst Rev.* 2006;3:CD005581.

Schwarz C, Volz A, Li C, Leucht S. Valproate for schizophrenia. *Cochrane Database Syst Rev.* 2008;(3):CD004028.

Whitehead C, Moss S, Cardno A, Lewis G. Antidepressants for people with both schizophrenia and depression. *Cochrane Database Syst Rev.* 2002;2:CD002305.

Polypharmacy

Barnes TR, Paton C. Antipsychotic polypharmacy in schizophrenia: benefits and risks. *CNS Drugs.* 2011;25:383-399.

Pregnancy and postpartum treatment

McCauley-Elsom K, Gurvich C, Elsom SJ, Kulkarni J. Antipsychotics in pregnancy. *J Psychiatr Ment Health Nurs.* 2010;17:97-104.

Solari H, Dickson KE, Miller L. Understanding and treating women with schizophrenia during pregnancy and postpartum – Motherisk Update 2008. *Can J Clin Pharmacol.* 2009;16:23-32.

Webb RT, Howard L, Abel KM. Antipsychotic drugs for non-affective psychosis during pregnancy and postpartum. *Cochrane Database Syst Rev.* 2004;(2):CD002305.

Psychosocial treatments

Overview

Dixon LB, Dickerson F, Bellack AS, et al. The 2009 schizophrenia PORT psychosocial treatment recommendations and summary statements. *Schizophr Bull.* 2010;36:48-70.

Huxley NA, Rendall M, Sederer L. Psychosocial treatments in schizophrenia: a review of the past 20 years. *J Nerv Ment Dis.* 2000;188:187-201.

Lysaker PH, Glynn SM, Wilkniss SM, Silverstein SM. Psychotherapy and recovery from schizophrenia: A review of potential applications and need for future study. *Psychol Serv.* 2010;7:75-91.

Taylor TL, Killaspy H, Wright C, et al. A systematic review of the international published literature relating to quality of institutional care for people with longer term mental health problems. *BMC Psychiatry.* 2009;9:55.

Cognitive behavior therapy

Huxley NA, Rendall M, Sederer L. Psychosocial treatments in schizophrenia: a review of the past 20 years. *J Nerv Ment Dis.* 2000;188:187-201.

Jackson HJ, McGorry PD, Killackey E, et al. Acute-phase and 1-year follow-up results of a randomized controlled trial of CBT versus befriending for first-episode psychosis: the ACE project. *Psychol Med.* 2008;38:725-735.

Jones C, Cormac I, Silveira da Mota Neto JI, Campbell C. Cognitive behaviour therapy for schizophrenia. *Cochrane Database Syst Rev.* 2004;(4):CD000524.

Sarin F, Wallin L, Widerlöv B. Cognitive behavior therapy for schizophrenia: a meta-analytical review of randomized controlled trials. *Nord J Psychiatry.* 2011;65:162-174.

Tarrier N, Yusupoff L, Kinney C, et al. Randomised controlled trial of intensive cognitive behaviour therapy for patients with chronic schizophrenia. *BMJ.* 1998; 317:303-307.

Day care

Marshall M, Crowther R, Almaraz-Serrano A, et al. Systematic reviews of the effectiveness of day care for people with severe mental disorders: (1) acute day hospital versus admission; (2) vocational rehabilitation; (3) day hospital versus outpatient care. *Health Technol Assess.* 2001;5:1-75.

Shek E, Stein AT, Shansis FM, Marshall M, Crowther R, Tyrer P. Day hospital versus outpatient care for people with schizophrenia. *Cochrane Database Syst Rev.* 2009;(4):CD003240.

Family interventions

Onwumere J, Bebbington P, Kuipers E. Family interventions in early psychosis: specificity and effectiveness. *Epidemiol Psychiatr Sci.* 2011;20:113-119.
Pharoah F, Mari J, Rathbone J, Wong W. Family intervention for schizophrenia. *Cochrane Database Syst Rev.* 2010;(12):CD000088.

Intensive case management

Dieterich M, Irving CB, Park B, Marshall M. Intensive case management for severe mental illness. *Cochrane Database Syst Rev.* 2010;(10):CD007906.

Integrated care including assertive community treatment

Lambert M, Bock T, Schöttle D, et al. Assertive community treatment as part of integrated care versus standard care: a 12-month trial in patients with first- and multiple-episode schizophrenia spectrum disorders treated with quetiapine immediate release (ACCESS trial). *J Clin Psychiatry.* 2010;71:1313-1323.
Petersen L, Jeppesen P, Thorup A, et al. A randomised multicenter trial of integrated versus standard treatment for patients with a first episode of psychotic illness. *BMJ.* 2005;331:602.
Weinmann S, Roick C, Martin L, Willich S, Becker T. Development of a set of schizophrenia quality indicators for integrated care. *Epidemiol Psychiatr Soc.* 2010;19:52-62.

Psychoeducation

Xia J, Merinder LB, Belgamwar MR. Psychoeducation for schizophrenia. *Cochrane Database Syst Rev.* 2011;(6):CD002831.
Rummel-Kluge C, Kissling W. Psychoeducation in schizophrenia: new developments and approaches in the field. *Curr Opin Psychiatry.* 2008;21:168-172.

Supportive therapy

Buckley LA, Pettit T, Adams CE. Supportive therapy for schizophrenia. *Cochrane Database Syst Rev.* 2007;(3):CD004716.

Vocational interventions

Crowther R, Marshall M, Bond G, Huxley P. Vocational rehabilitation for people with severe mental illness. *Cochrane Database Syst Rev.* 2001;(2):CD003080.
Killackey E, Jackson HJ, McGorry PD. Vocational intervention in first-episode psychosis: individual placement and support v. treatment as usual. *Br J Psychiatry.* 2008;193:114-120.
Marwaha S, Johnson S. Schizophrenia and employment: A review. *Soc Psychiatry Psychiatr Epidemiol.* 2004;39:337-349.
Tsang HW, Leung AY, Chung RC, Bell M, Cheung WM. Review on vocational predictors: a systematic review of predictors of vocational outcomes among individuals with schizophrenia: an update since 1998. *Aust N Z J Psychiatry.* 2010;44:495-504.

Relapse prevention

Gleeson JF, Alvarez-Jimenez M, Cotton SM, Parker AG, Hetrick S. A systematic review of relapse measurement in randomized controlled trials of relapse prevention in first-episode psychosis. *Schizophr Res*. 2010;119:79-88.

Remission and recovery

Remission

Andreasen NC, Carpenter WT Jr, Kane JM, Lasser RA, Marder SR, Weinberger DR. Remission in schizophrenia: proposed criteria and rationale for consensus. *Am J Psychiatry*. 2005;162:441-449.

Kane JM. An evidence-based strategy for remission in schizophrenia. *J Clin Psychiatry* 2008;69(suppl 3):25-30.

Lambert M, Naber D, Schacht A, et al. Predicting remission and recovery in 392 never-treated patients with schizophrenia. *Acta Psychiatr Scand*. 2008;118:220-229.

Lambert M, Karow A, Leucht S, Schimmelmann BG, Naber D. Remission in schizophrenia: its validity, frequency, predictors and patients' perspective 5 years after. *Dialogues Clin Neurosci*. 2010;12:393-407.

Recovery

Harrison G, Hopper K, Craig T, et al. Recovery from psychotic illness: a 15- and 25-year international follow-up study. *Br J Psychiatry*. 2001;178:506-517.

Hegarty JD, Baldessarini RJ, Tohen M, Waternaux C, Oepen G. One hundred years of schizophrenia: a meta-analysis of the outcome literature. *Am J Psychiatry*. 1994;151:1409-1416.

Lambert M, Schimmelmann BG, Schacht A, et al. Long-term patterns of subjective wellbeing in schizophrenia: cluster, predictors of cluster affiliation, and their relation to recovery criteria in 2842 patients followed over 3 years. *Schizophr Res*. 2009;107:165-172.

Resnick SG, Fontana A, Lehman AF, Rosenheck RA. An empirical conceptualization of the recovery orientation. *Schizophr Res*. 2005;75:119-128.

Schizophrenia guidelines

American Psychiatric Association. *Practice Guideline for the Treatment of Patients with Schizophrenia*, 2nd compendium. Arlington, VA: APA, 2004.

Falkai P, Wobrock T, Lieberman J, Glenthoj B, Gattaz WF, Moller HJ, WFSBP Task Force on Treatment Guidelines for Schizophrenia. World Federation of Societies of Biological Psychiatry (WFSBP) guidelines for biological treatment of schizophrenia, Part 1: acute treatment of schizophrenia. *World J Biol Psychiatry*. 2005;6:132-191.

Lehman AF, Kreyenbuhl J, Buchanan RW, et al. The Schizophrenia Patient Outcomes Research Team (PORT): updated treatment recommendations 2003. *Schizophr Bull*. 2004;30:193-217.

National Institute for Health and Clinical Excellence (NICE). *Schizophrenia. Core interventions in the treatment and management of schizophrenia in primary and secondary care*. Clinical Guideline 1, National Collaborating Centre for Mental Health. London, UK: NICE; 2002.

Royal Australian and New Zealand College of Psychiatrists. Royal Australian and New Zealand College of Psychiatrists clinical practice guidelines for the treatment of schizophrenia and related disorders. *Aust NZ J Psychiatry*. 2005;39:1-30.

Shared decision-making and motivational interviewing

Duncan E, Best C, Hagen S. Shared decision making interventions for people with mental health conditions. *Cochrane Database Syst Rev.* 2010;(1):CD007297.

Makoul G, Clayman ML. An integrative model of shared decision making in medical encounters. *Patient Educ Couns.* 2006;60:301-312.

Miller CE, Johnson JL. Motivational interviewing. *Can Nurse.* 2001;97:32-33.

Miller WR, Rollnick S. *Motivational Interviewing: Preparing People for Change.* New York, NY: The Guilford Press; 1999.

Tibaldi G, Salvador-Carulla L, García-Gutierrez JC. From treatment adherence to advanced shared decision making: new professional strategies and attitudes in mental health care. *Curr Clin Pharmacol.* 2011;6:91-99.

Side effects

Overview

Edwards SJ, Smith CJ. Tolerability of atypical antipsychotics in the treatment of adults with schizophrenia or bipolar disorder: a mixed treatment comparison of randomized controlled trials. *Clin Ther.* 2009;31:1345-1359.

Sharif Z. Side effects as influencers of treatment outcome. *J Clin Psychiatry.* 2008;69(suppl 3):38-43.

Cardiological side effects

De Hert M, Vancampfort D, Correll CU, et al. Guidelines for screening and monitoring of cardiometabolic risk in schizophrenia: systematic evaluation. *Br J Psychiatry.* 2011;199:99-105.

De Hert M, Detraux J, van Winkel R, Yu W, Correll CU. Metabolic and cardiovascular adverse effects associated with antipsychotic drugs. *Nat Rev Endocrinol.* 2011;8:114-126.

Del Rosario ME, Weachter R, Flaker GC. Drug-induced QT prolongation and sudden death. *Mo Med.* 2010;107:53-58.

Glassman AH, Bigger JT Jr. Antipsychotic drugs: prolonged QTc interval, torsade de pointes, and sudden death. *Am J Psychiatry.* 2001;158:1774-1782.

Meltzer HY, Davidson M, Glassman AH, Vieweg WV. Assessing cardiovascular risks versus clinical benefits of atypical antipsychotic drug treatment. *J Clin Psychiatry.* 2002;63(suppl 9):25-29.

Diabetes

Sernyak MJ, Leslie DL, Alarcon RD, Losonczy MF, Rosenheck R. Association of diabetes mellitus with use of atypical neuroleptics in the treatment of schizophrenia. *Am J Psychiatry.* 2002;159:561-566.

Smith M, Hopkins D, Peveler RC, Holt RI, Woodward M, Ismail K. First- v. second-generation antipsychotics and risk for diabetes in schizophrenia: systematic review and meta-analysis. *Br J Psychiatry.* 2008;192:406-411.

Extrapyramidal side effects

Gao K, Kemp DE, Ganocy SJ, Gajwani P, Xia G, Calabrese JR. Antipsychotic-induced extrapyramidal side effects in bipolar disorder and schizophrenia: a systematic review. *J Psychopharmacol.* 2008;28:203-209.

Kane JM, Fleischhacker WW, Hansen L, et al. Akathisia: an updated review focusing on second-generation antipsychotics. *J Clin Psychiatry.* 2009;70:627-643.

Remington G, Bezchlibnyk-Butler K. Management of acute antipsychotic-induced extrapyramidal syndromes. *CNS Drugs.* 1996;5(suppl 1):21-35.

Rummel-Kluge C, Komossa K, Schwarz S, et al. Second-generation antipsychotic drugs and extrapyramidal side effects: a systematic review and meta-analysis of head-to-head comparisons. *Schizophr Bull.* 2012;38:167-177.

Metabolic side effects

Monteleone P, Martiadis V, Maj M. Management of schizophrenia with obesity, metabolic, and endocrinological disorders. *Psychiatr Clin North Am.* 2009;32:775-794.

Newcomer JW. Second-generation (atypical) antipsychotics and metabolic effects. *CNS Drugs.* 2005;19(suppl 1):1-93.

Rummel-Kluge C, Komossa K, Schwarz S, et al. Head-to-head comparisons of metabolic side effects of second generation antipsychotics in the treatment of schizophrenia: a systematic review and meta-analysis. *Schizophr Res.* 2010;123:225-233.

Sexual dysfunctions including hyperprolactinemia

Berner MM, Hagen M, Kriston L. Management of sexual dysfunction due to antipsychotic drug therapy. *Cochrane Database Syst Rev.* 2007;(1):CD003546.

Bushe C, Shaw M, Peveler RC. A review of the association between antipsychotic use and hyperprolactinaemia. *J Psychopharmacol.* 2008;22:46-45.

Citrome L. Current guidelines and their recommendations for prolactin monitoring in psychosis. *J Psychopharmacol.* 2008;22:90-97.

Dursun SM, Wildgust HJ, Strickland P, Goodwin GM, Citrome L, Lean M. The emerging physical health challenges of antipsychotic associated hyperprolactinaemia in patients with serious mental illness. *J Psychopharmacol.* 2008;22:3-5.

Henderson DC, Doraiswamy PM. Prolactin-related and metabolic adverse effects of atypical antipsychotic agents. *J Clin Psychiatry.* 2008;69(suppl 1):32-44.

Holt RI. Medical causes and consequences of hyperprolactinaemia. A context for psychiatrists. *J Psychopharmacol.* 2008;22:28-37.

Inder WJ, Castle D. Antipsychotic-induced hyperprolactinaemia. *Aust N Z J Psychiatry.* 2011;45:830-837.

Peveler RC, Branford D, Citrome L, et al. Antipsychotics and hyperprolactinaemia: clinical recommendations. *J Psychopharmacol.* 2008;22:98-103.

Smith SM. The impact of hyperprolactinaemia on sexual function in patients with psychosis. *J Psychopharmacol.* 2008;22:63-69.

Walters J, Jones I. Clinical questions and uncertainty – prolactin measurement in patients with schizophrenia and bipolar disorder. *J Psychopharmacol.* 2008;22:82-89.

Tardive dyskinesia

American Psychiatric Association Task Force on Tardive Dyskinesia. *Tardive Dyskinesia: A Task Force Report of the American Psychiatric Association.* Washington, DC: APA, 1992.

Bergen J, Kitchin R, Berry G. Predictors of the course of tardive dyskinesia in patients receiving neuroleptics. *Biol Psychiatry.* 1992;32:580-594.

Correll CU, Schenk EM. Tardive dyskinesia and new antipsychotics. *Curr Opin Psychiatry.* 2008;21:151-156.

Correll CU, Leucht S, Kane JM. Lower risk for tardive dyskinesia associated with second-generation antipsychotics: a systematic review of 1-year studies. *Am J Psychiatry*. 2004;161:414-425.

Schooler NR, Kane JM. Research diagnoses for tardive dyskinesia. *Arch Gen Psychiatry*. 1982;39:486-487.

Tarsy D, Lungu C, Baldessarini RJ. Epidemiology of tardive dyskinesia before and during the era of modern antipsychotic drugs. *Handb Clin Neurol*. 2011;100:601-616.

Tenback DE, van Harten PN, van Os J. Non-therapeutic risk factors for onset of tardive dyskinesia in schizophrenia: a meta-analysis. *Mov Disord*. 2009;24:2309-2315.

Weight gain

Alvarez-Jiménez M, Hetrick SE, González-Blanch C, Gleeson JF, McGorry PD. Non-pharmacological management of antipsychotic-induced weight gain: systematic review and meta-analysis of randomized controlled trials. *Br J Psychiatry*. 2008;193:101-107.

American Diabetes Association, American Psychiatric Association, American Association of Clinical Endocrinologists, North American Association for the Study of Obesity. Consensus development conference on antipsychotic drugs and obesity and diabetes. *Diabetes Care*. 2004;27:596-601.

De Hert M, van Winkel R, Van Eyck D, et al. Prevalence of diabetes, metabolic syndrome and metabolic abnormalities in schizophrenia over the course of the illness: a cross-sectional study. *Clin Pract Epidemiol Ment Health*. 2006;2:14-26.

Faulkner G, Cohn T, Remington G. Interventions to reduce weight gain in schizophrenia. *Cochrane Database Syst Rev*. 2007;(1):CD005148.

Lett TA, Wallace TJ, Chowdhury NI, Tiwari AK, Kennedy JL, Müller DJ. Pharmacogenetics of antipsychotic-induced weight gain: review and clinical implications. *Mol Psychiatry*. 2012. In press.

Megna JL, Schwartz TL, Siddiqui UA, Herrera Rojas M. Obesity in adults with serious and persistent mental illness: a review of postulated mechanisms and current interventions. *Ann Clin Psychiatry*. 2011;23:131-140.

Somatic diseases

Marder SR, Essock SM, Miller AL, et al. Physical health monitoring of patients with schizophrenia. *Am J Psychiatry*. 2004;161:1334-1349.

Oud MJ, Meyboom-de Jong B. Somatic diseases in patients with schizophrenia in general practice: their prevalence and health care. *BMC Fam Pract*. 2009;10:32.

Saha S, Chant D, McGrath J. A systematic review of mortality in schizophrenia: is the differential mortality gap worsening over time? *Arch Gen Psychiatry*. 2007;64:1123-1131.

Substance use disorders

Baker A, Bucci S, Lewin TJ, Kay-Lambkin F, Constable PM, Carr VJ. Cognitive-behavioural therapy for substance use disorders in people with psychotic disorders: Randomised controlled trial. *Br J Psychiatry*. 2006;188:439-448.

Barrowclough C, Haddock G, Wykes T, et al. Integrated motivational interviewing and cognitive behavioural therapy for people with psychosis and comorbid substance misuse: randomised controlled trial. *BMJ*. 2010;341:6325.

Barrowclough C, Haddock G, Tarrier N, et al. Randomized controlled trial of motivational interviewing, cognitive behavior therapy, and family intervention for patients with comorbid schizophrenia and substance use disorders. *Am J Psychiatry*. 2001;158:1706-1713.

Bellack AS, Bennett ME, Gearon JS, Brown CH, Yang Y. A randomized clinical trial of a new behavioral treatment for drug abuse in people with severe and persistent mental illness. *Arch Gen Psychiatry*. 2006;63:426-432.

Blanchard JJ, Brown SA, Horan WP, Sherwood AR. Substance use disorders in schizophrenia: review, integration, and a proposed model. *Clin Psychol Rev*. 2000;20:207-234.

Cleary M, Hunt G, Matheson S, Siegfried N, Walter G. Psychosocial interventions for people with both severe mental illness and substance misuse. *Cochrane Database Syst Rev*. 2008;(1):CD001088.

Denis C, Lavie E, Fatséas M, Auriacombe M. Psychotherapeutic interventions for cannabis abuse and/or dependence in outpatient settings. *Cochrane Database Syst Rev*. 2006;(3):CD005336.

Drake RE, O'Neal EL, Wallach MA. A systematic review of psychosocial research on psychosocial interventions for people with co-occurring severe mental and substance use disorders. *J Sub Abuse Treat*. 2008;34:123-138.

Edwards J, Elkins K, Hinton M, et al. Randomized controlled trial of a cannabis-focused intervention for young people with first-episode psychosis. *Acta Psychiatr Scand*. 2006;114:109-117.

Green AI, Noordsy DL, Brunette MF, O'Keefe C. Substance abuse and schizophrenia: pharmacotherapeutic intervention. *J Subst Abuse Treat*. 2008;34:61-71.

Haddock G, Barrowclough C, Tarrier N, et al. Cognitive-behavioural therapy and motivational intervention for schizophrenia and substance misuse: 18-month outcomes of a randomised controlled trial. *Br J Psychiatry*. 2003;183:418-426.

Hjorthøj C, Fohlmann A, Nordentoft M. Treatment of cannabis use disorders in people with schizophrenia spectrum disorders – a systematic review. *Addict Behav*. 2009;34:520-525.

Koskinen J, Löhönen J, Koponen H, Isohanni M, Miettunen J. Rate of cannabis use disorders in clinical samples of patients with schizophrenia: a meta-analysis. *Schizophr Bull*. 2010;36:1115-1130.

Lambert M, Conus P, Lubman DI, et al. The impact of substance use disorders on clinical outcome in 643 patients with first-episode psychosis. *Acta Psychiatr Scand*. 2005;112:141-148.

Regier DA, Farmer ME, Rae DS, et al. Comorbidity of mental disorders with alcohol and other drug abuse: results from the Epidemiologic Catchment Area (ECA) Study. *JAMA*. 1990;264:2511-2518.

Suicidal behavior

Bowers L, Banda T, Nijman H. Suicide inside: a systematic review of inpatient suicides. *J Nerv Ment Dis*. 2010;198:315-328.

Caldwell CB, Gottesman II. Schizophrenics kill themselves too: a review of risk factors for suicide. *Schizophr Bull*. 1990;16:571-589.

Hawton K, Sutton L, Haw C, Sinclair J, Deeks JJ. Schizophrenia and suicide: systematic review of risk factors. *Br J Psychiatry*. 2005;187:9-20.

Kasckow J, Felmet K, Zisook S. Managing suicide risk in patients with schizophrenia. *CNS Drugs*. 2011;25:129-143.

Mamo DC. Managing suicidality in schizophrenia. *Can J Psychiatry*. 2007;52(suppl 1):59-70.

Meltzer HY, Alphs L, Green AI, et al, International Suicide Prevention Trial Study Group. Clozapine treatment for suicidality in schizophrenia: International Suicide Prevention Trial (InterSePT). *Arch Gen Psychiatry*. 2003;60:82-91.

Switching antipsychotics

Correll CU. Switching and combining antipsychotics. *CNS Spectr*. 2010;15 (suppl 6): 8-11.

Mukundan A, Faulkner G, Cohn T, Remington G. Antipsychotic switching for people with schizophrenia who have neuroleptic-induced weight or metabolic problems. *Cochrane Database Syst Rev*. 2010;(12):CD006629.

Treatment-resistant schizophrenia

Barbui C, Signoretti A, Mulè S, Boso M, Cipriani A. Does the addition of a second antipsychotic drug improve clozapine treatment? *Schizophr Bull.* 2009;35:458-468.

Chakos M, Lieberman J, Hoffman E, Bradford D, Sheitman B. Effectiveness of second-generation antipsychotics in patients with treatment-resistant schizophrenia: a review and meta-analysis of randomized trials. *Am J Psychiatry.* 2001;158:518-526.

Elkis H. Treatment-resistant schizophrenia. *Psychiatr Clin North Am.* 2007;30:511-533.

Huber CG, Naber D, Lambert M. Incomplete remission and treatment resistance in first-episode psychosis: definition, prevalence and predictors. *Expert Opin Pharmacother.* 2008;12:2027-2038.

Lambert M, Naber D, Huber CG. Management of incomplete remission and treatment resistance in first-episode psychosis. *Expert Opin Pharmacother.* 2008;9:2039-2051.

McIlwain ME, Harrison J, Wheeler AJ, Russell BR. Pharmacotherapy for treatment-resistant schizophrenia. *Neuropsychiatr Dis Treat.* 2011;7:135-149.

Mouaffak F, Tranulis C, Gourevitch R, Augmentation strategies of clozapine with antipsychotics in the treatment of ultraresistant schizophrenia. *Clin Neuropharmacol.* 2006;29:28-33.

Nielsen J, Damkier P, Lublin H, Taylor D. Optimizing clozapine treatment. *Acta Psychiatr Scand.* 2011;123:411-422.

Pantelis C, Lambert TJ. Managing patients with "treatment-resistant" schizophrenia. *Med J Aust.* 2003;178(suppl):62-66.

Potkin SG, Bera R, Gulasekaram B, et al. Plasma clozapine concentrations predict clinical response in treatment-resistant schizophrenia. *J Clin Psychiatry.* 1994;55:133-136.

Remington G, Saha A, Chong SA, Shammi C. Augmenting strategies in clozapine-resistant schizophrenia. *CNS Drugs.* 2006;20:171-189.

Spina E, Avenoso A, Facciolà G, et al. Relationship between plasma concentrations of clozapine and norclozapine and therapeutic response in patients with schizophrenia resistant to conventional neuroleptics. *Psychopharmacology.* 2000;148:83-89.

Suzuki T, Remington G, Mulsant BH, et al. Treatment resistant schizophrenia and response to antipsychotics: a review. *Schizophr Res.* 2011;133:54-62.

Printed by Publishers' Graphics LLC
BCISO131121.15.22.1